Escape From Witch Castle
Take Another Mouthful Series

First Edition

Copyright © Take Another Media Ltd 2014

ISBN 978-0-9929052-1-7
Published in April 2014 by Take Another Media Ltd,
Publishers of the Take Another Mouthful Stories.

Story Sarah Gregory
Illustrations Dilara Arin
Photography Dave Nicholson

This ebook is copyright material and must not be copied, reproduced, transferred, distributed, leased, licensed or publicly performed or used in anyway except as specifically permitted in writing by the publishers, as allowed under the terms and conditions under which is was purchased or as strictly permitted by applicable copyright law. Any unauthorised distribution or use of this text may be a direct infringement of the author's and publisher's rights and those responsible may be liable in law accordingly.

The right of Take Another Media Ltd is to be identified as author of this work has been asserted by their accordance with sections 77 and 78 of the Copyright, Designs and Patents Act 1988.

All rights reserved. No part of this publication may be reproduced, stored in retrieval system, copied in any form or by any means, electronic, mechanical, photocopying, recording or otherwise transmitted without written permission from the publisher. You must not circulate this book in any format.

Take Another Media Limited Reg. No. 8885654

For Take Another Media Ltd Address please contact
sarah@takeanothermouthful.com

Escape From Witch Castle

Take Another Mouthful Series

Sarah Gregory

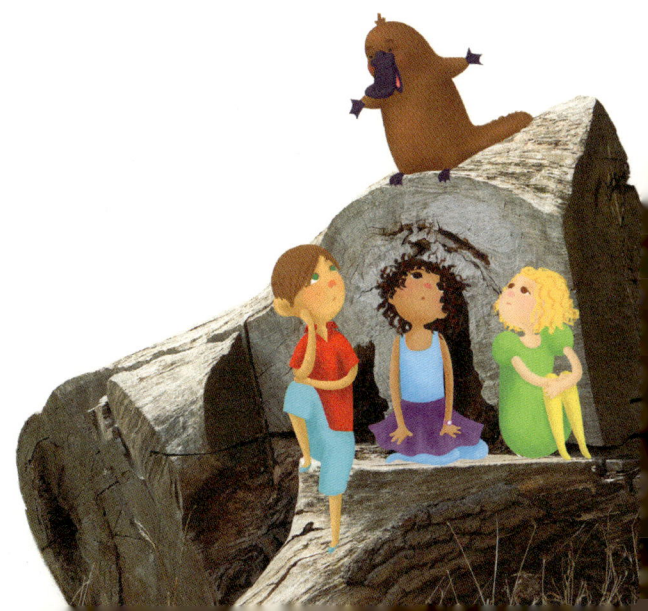

Contents

introduction	5
about us	6 - 7
story	8 - 45
hints & tips	46 - 47
about the author	48 - 49

Introduction
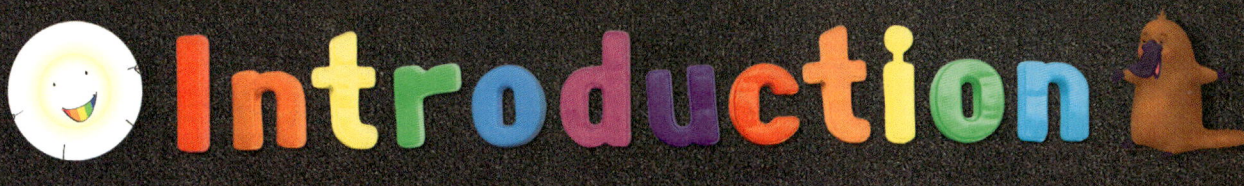

Take Another Mouthful
stories help create fun family mealtimes.

Encouraging children to eat, through adventures written for the their enjoyment. We always recommend mindful eating.

I'm a mother of four very different children so our stories are naturally flexible. We've allowed for missed mouthfuls, conversation and breaks.

Each story is written so you can pause long enough for your loved ones to chew and enjoy their food at a pace that is right for them.

We prefer quality rather than quantity when it comes to mealtimes. Quality food, Quality time and Quality fun!

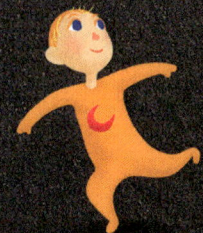
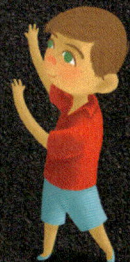

Visit www.takeanothermouthful.com for a great selection of Take Another Mouthful recipes for fantastic dinners, and also grown up, but useful links to UK guidelines on portion sizes and much more.

Take Another Mouthful stories are intended to help make mealtimes fun but are not a substitute for professional guidance, if you feel your child has deeper issues with food or is unwell please contact the relevant health professionals in your area.

Take Another Mouthful was born when my husband Fergus was a wee nipper and refused to eat at mealtimes. His parents despaired as many parents do.

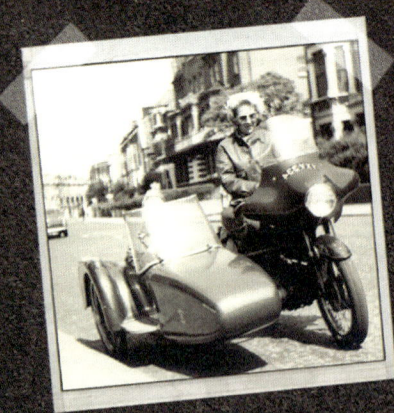

His Granny, Emily, was an adventurous character and had a different, we like to think revolutionary, solution.

Emily had a flair for telling stories full of mystery, humour and adventure, so she brought them to the dinner table.

Fergus would have been labelled a 'classic fussy eater' when he was a child.

As a direct result of his Granny's stories he has fond memories of his mealtime experiences and grew into an adult with a love of food and fine stories.

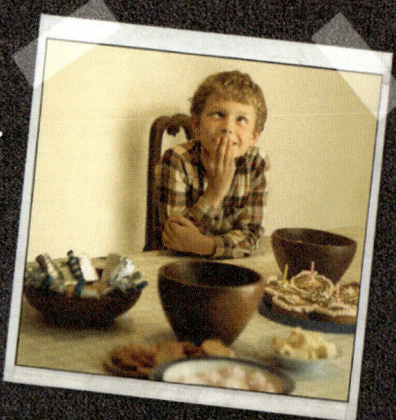

It was Fergus' Mum, now Granny Erica, who first introduced me to Take Another Mouthful stories when our then young son Thomas started refusing to eat dinner.

We were naturally very worried and stressed. As a Mum I wanted to change Thomas' relationship with food in a healthy and happy way.

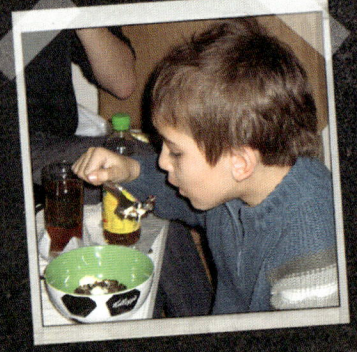

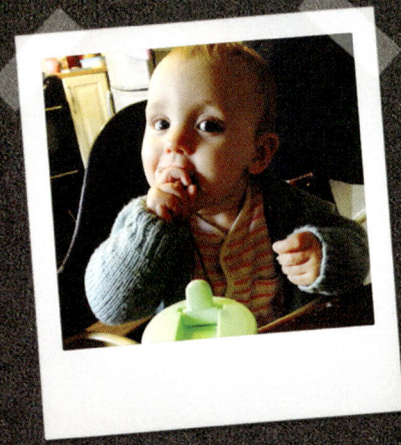

Since then we have had three more children and the stories have worked amazingly in different ways, but always Take Another Mouthful stories have helped create fun family mealtimes.

We feel its time to share our secret with the world and so here it is, our first Take Another Mouthful book.

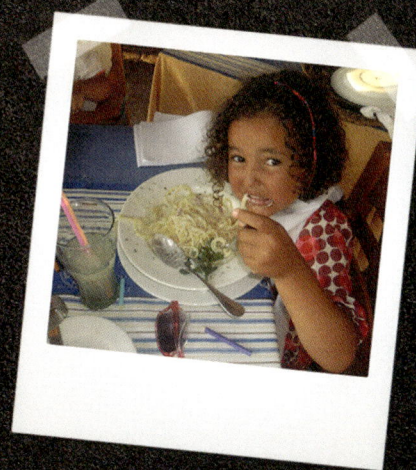

We hope you find it useful and fun! As Granny Emily first said, 'Come on! There's Adventure after every Mouthful!'

Thanks for reading,

Sarah xx

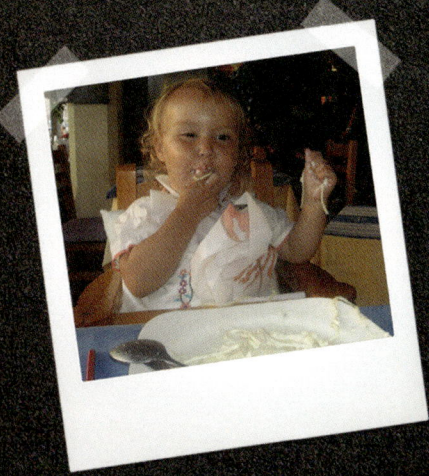

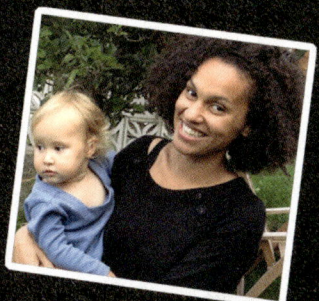

PS we'd love to hear your experiences with Take Another Mouthful stories...

...please stay in touch at www.takeanothermouthful.com

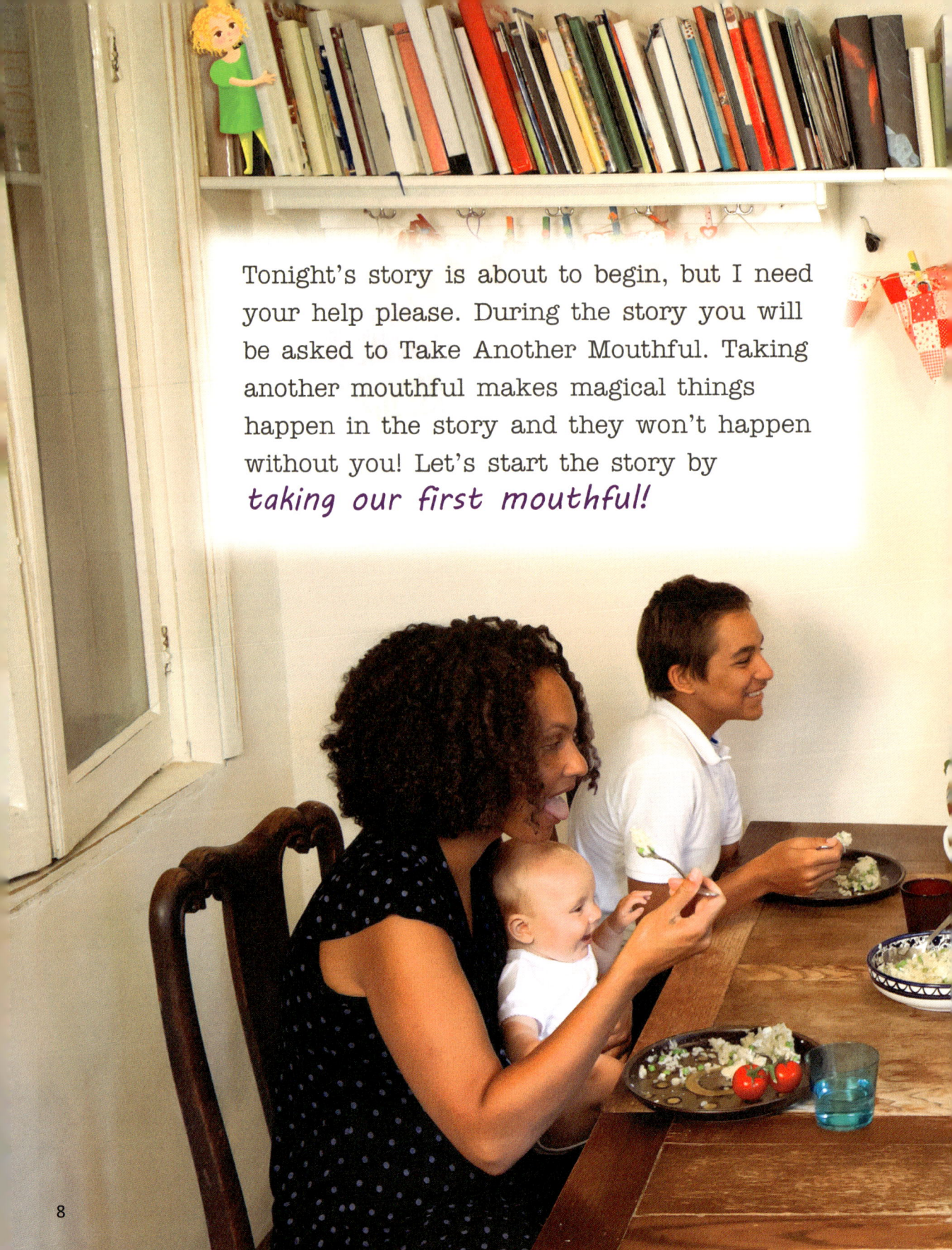

Tonight's story is about to begin, but I need your help please. During the story you will be asked to Take Another Mouthful. Taking another mouthful makes magical things happen in the story and they won't happen without you! Let's start the story by *taking our first mouthful!*

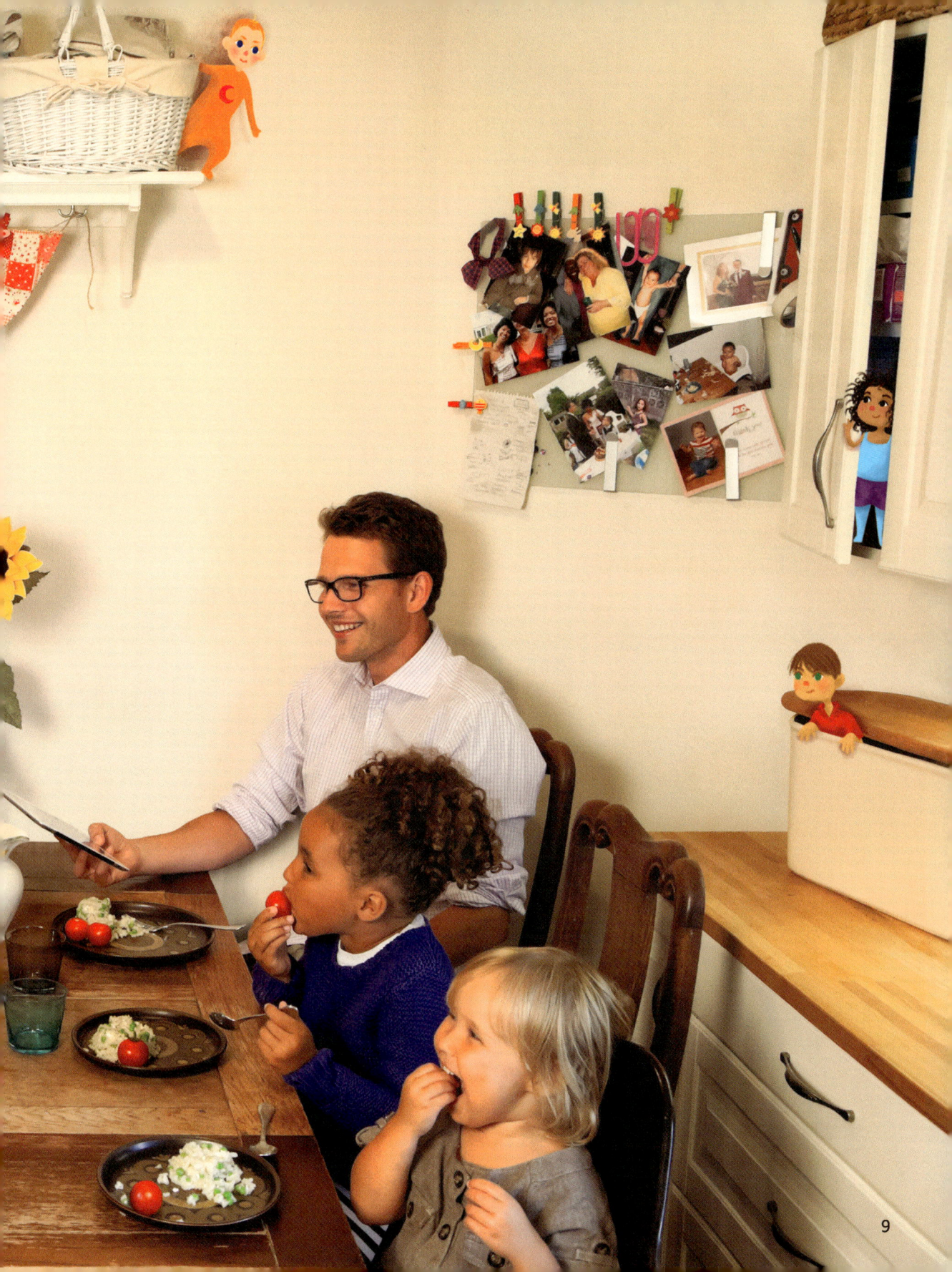

Edith and Thomas were riding their scooters to the park to meet their two sisters Agnes and Amelie. The sun was shining and the birds were singing in the trees. When they arrived at the entrance to the park the clouds in the sky turned grey and looked angry... If you want to find out what was about to happen, you need to *take another mouthful!*

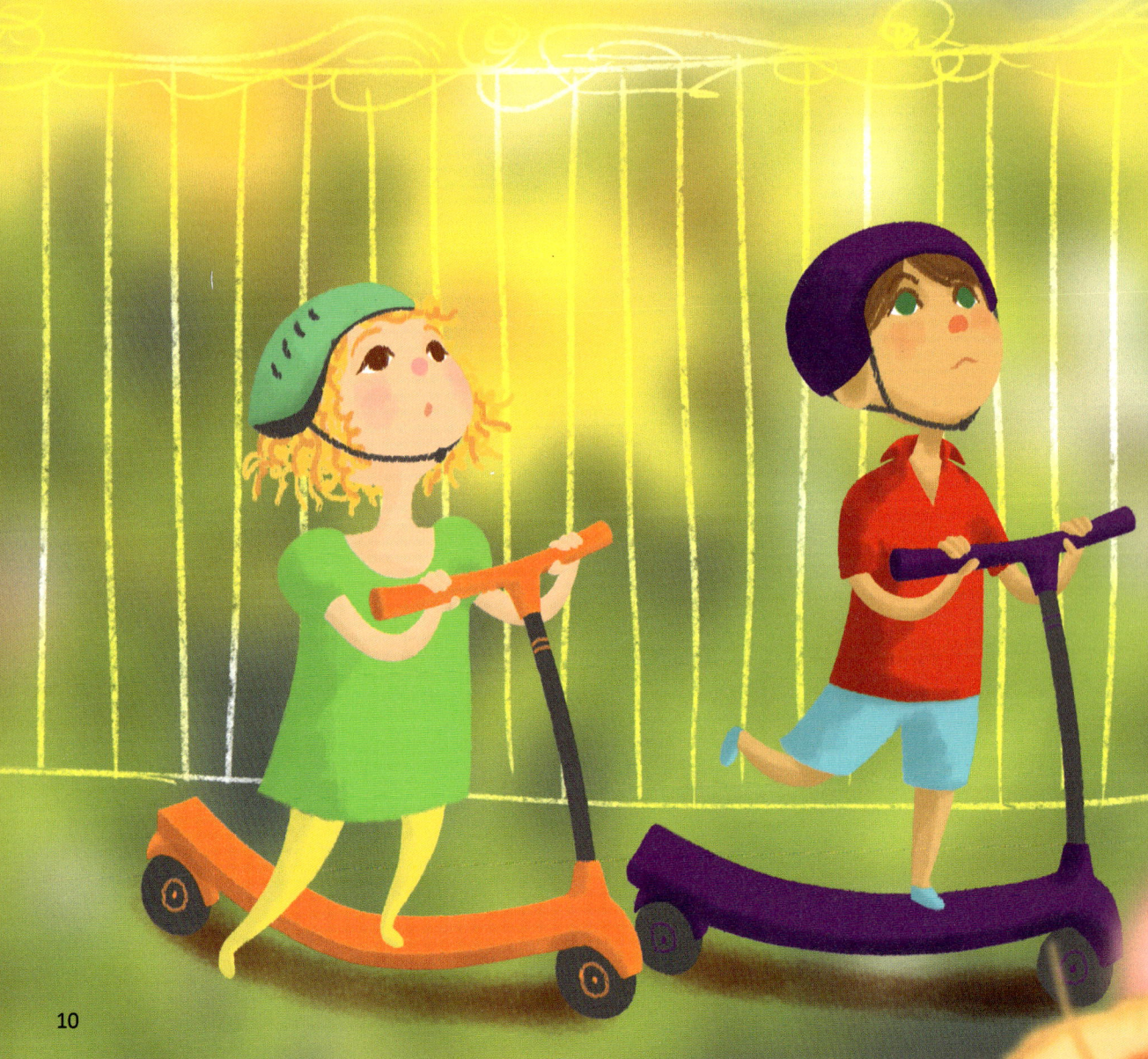

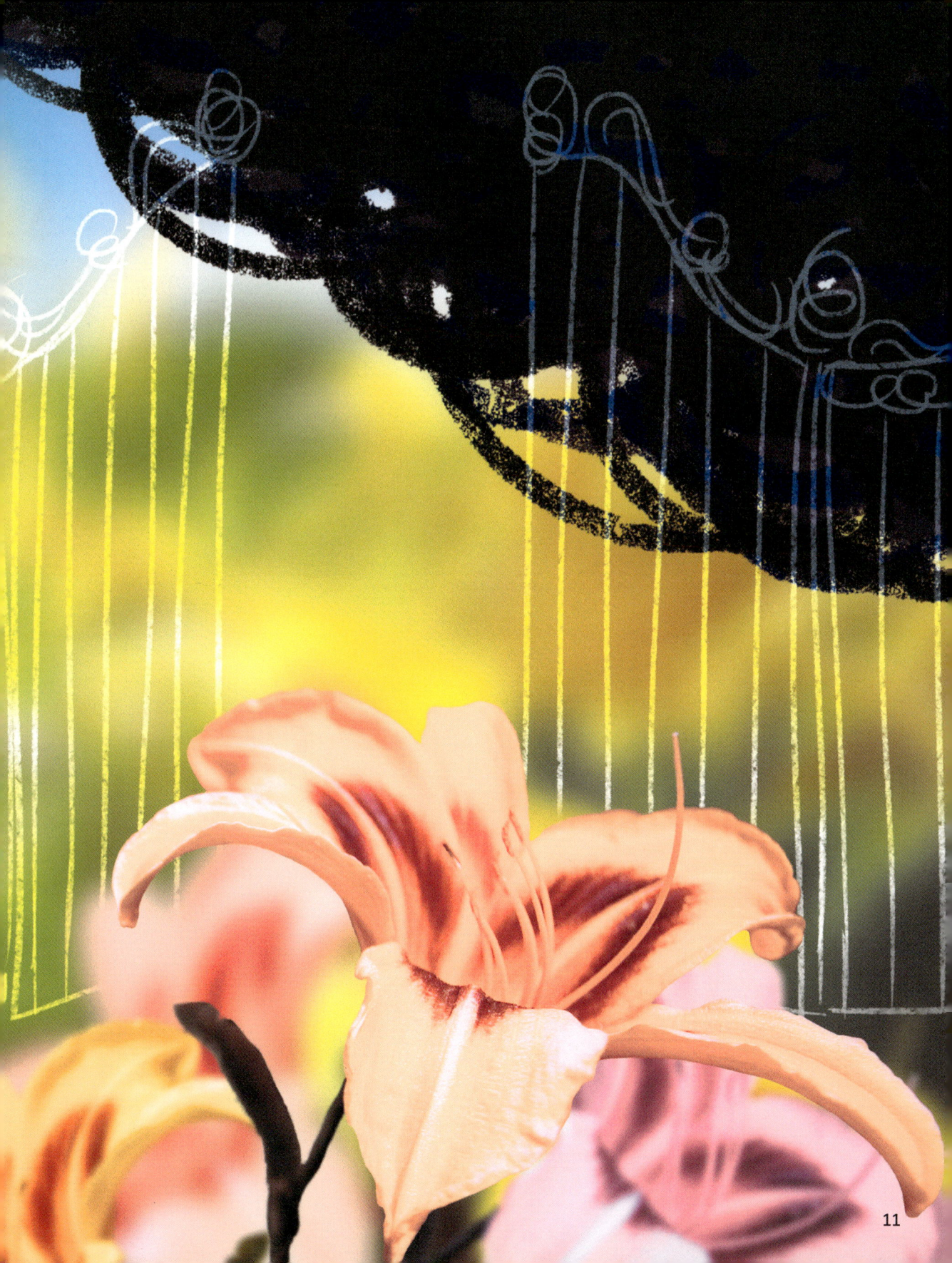

A swirling, whirling tornado appeared over the park sucking the swings, the slide and their favourite roundabout into the air! This was no ordinary storm. The children gasped as they saw the cloud was full of wicked witches on flying broomsticks! The witches were heading straight for them. Your friends need courage, quickly! *Take another mouthful!*

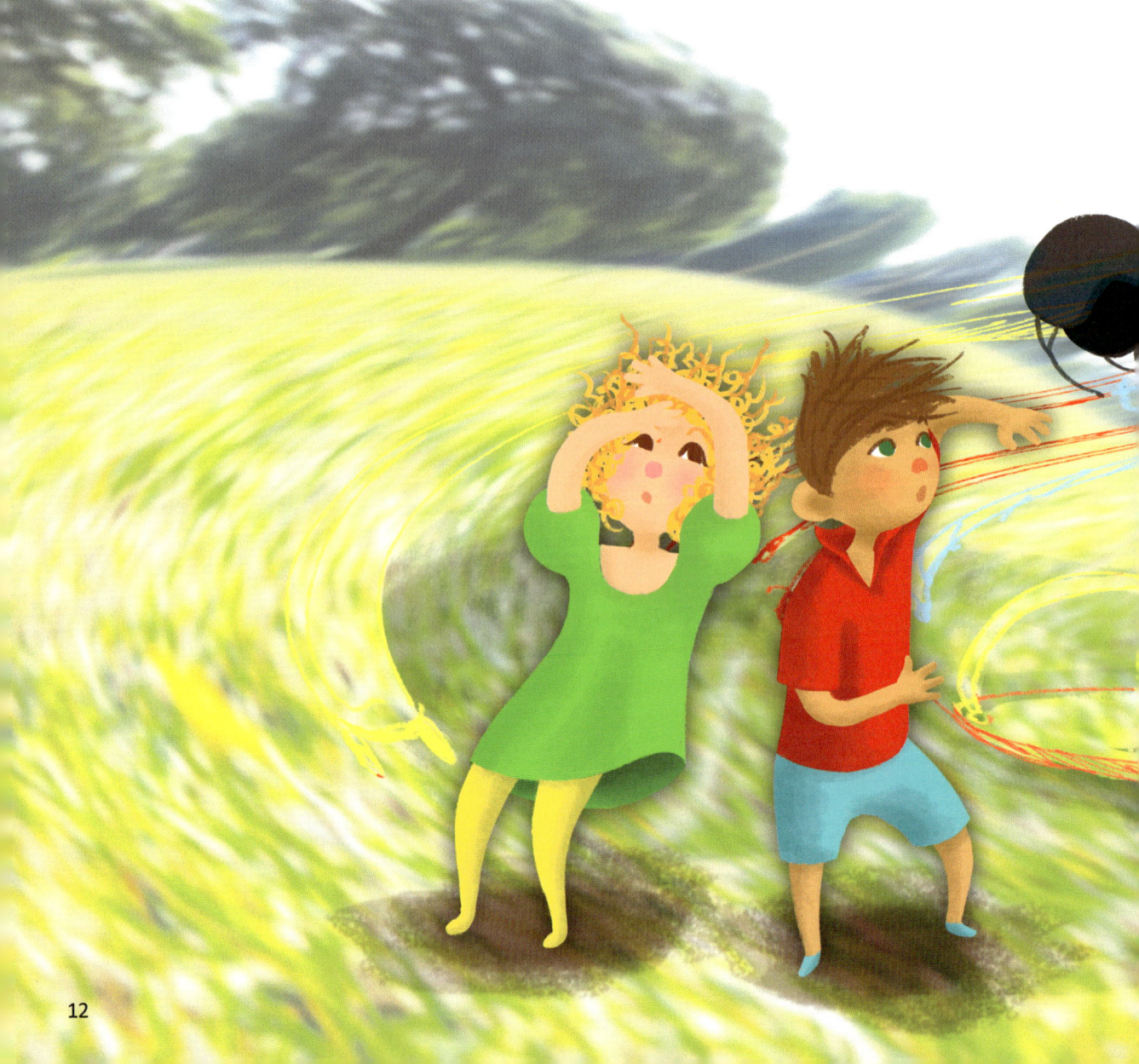

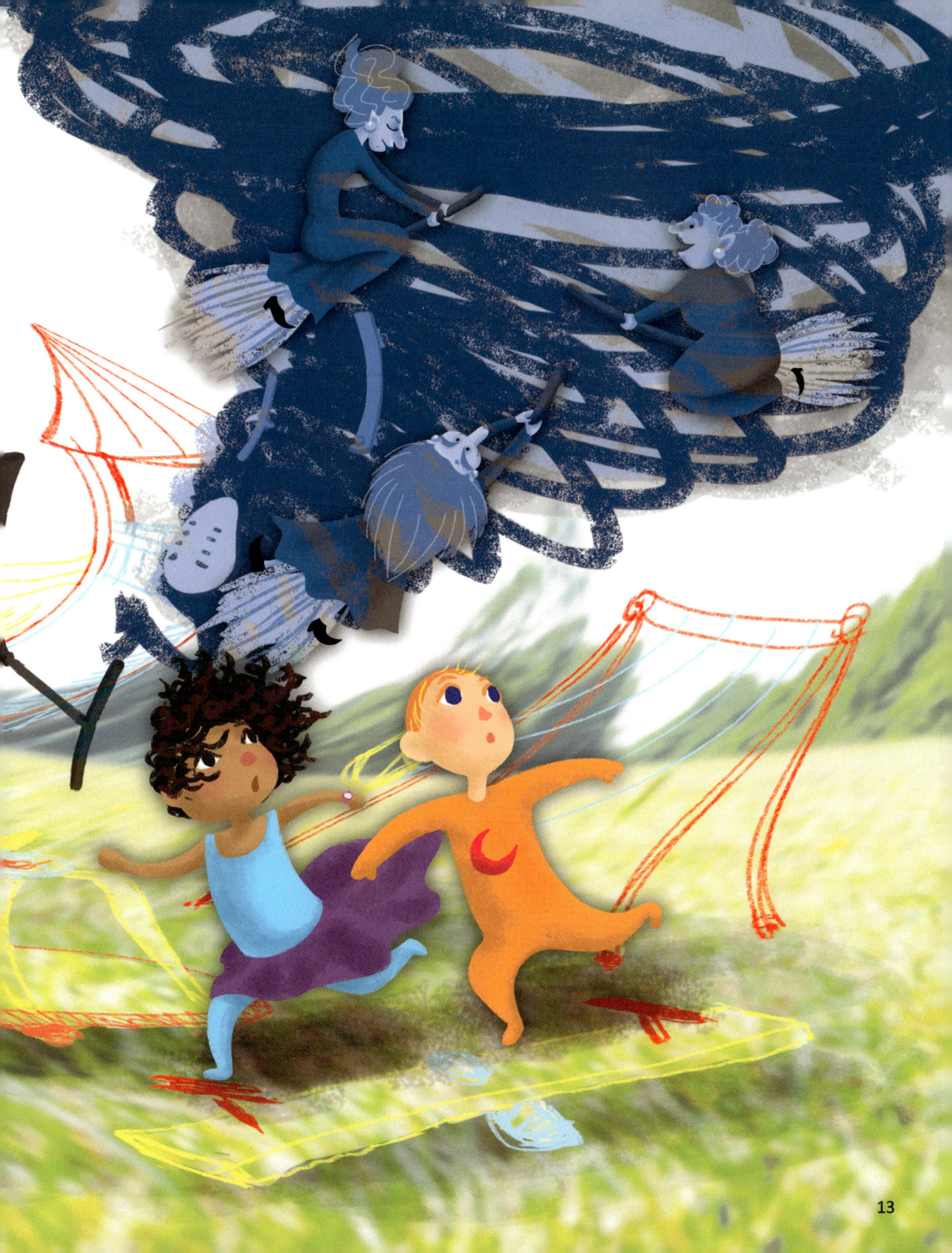

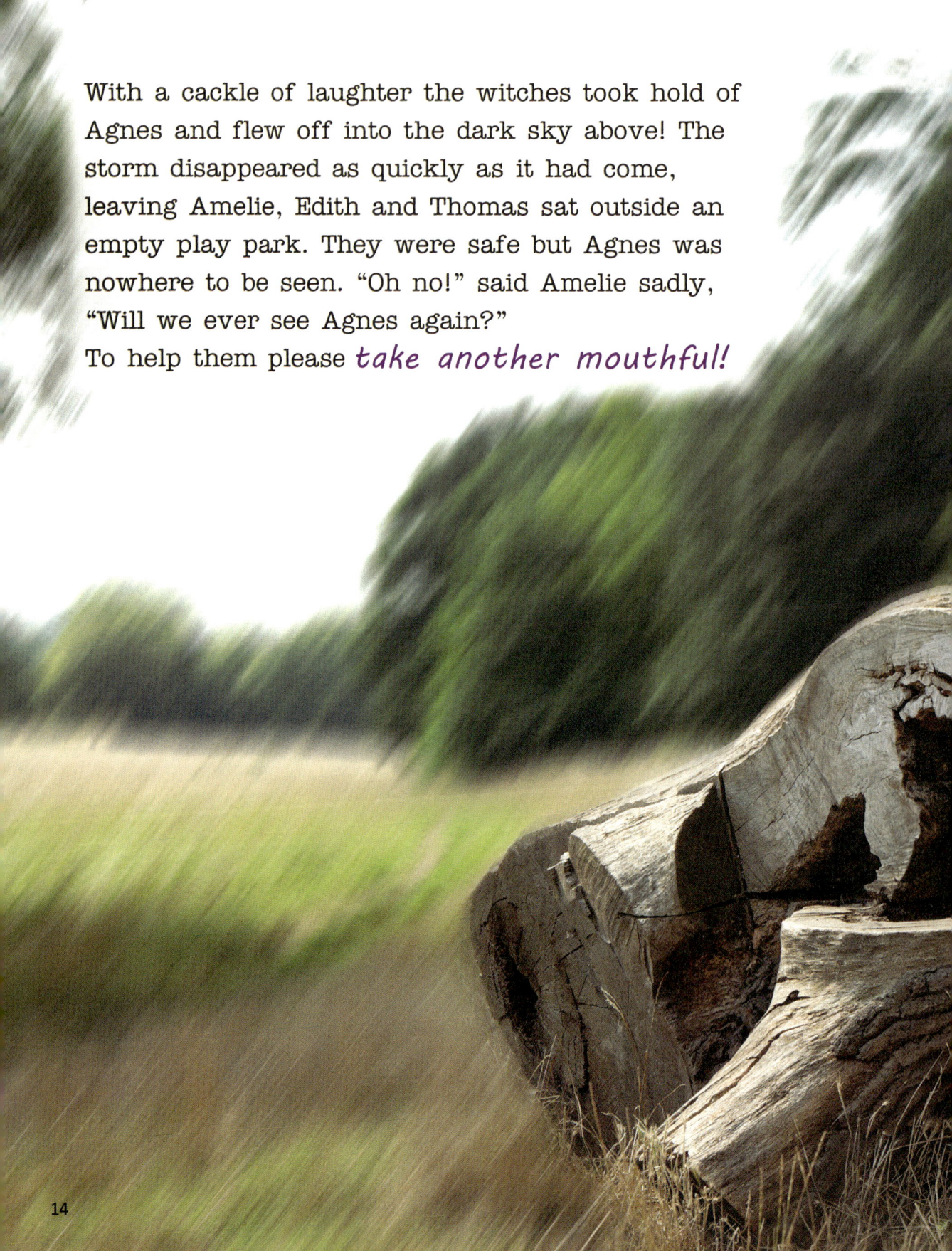

With a cackle of laughter the witches took hold of Agnes and flew off into the dark sky above! The storm disappeared as quickly as it had come, leaving Amelie, Edith and Thomas sat outside an empty play park. They were safe but Agnes was nowhere to be seen. "Oh no!" said Amelie sadly, "Will we ever see Agnes again?"
To help them please *take another mouthful!*

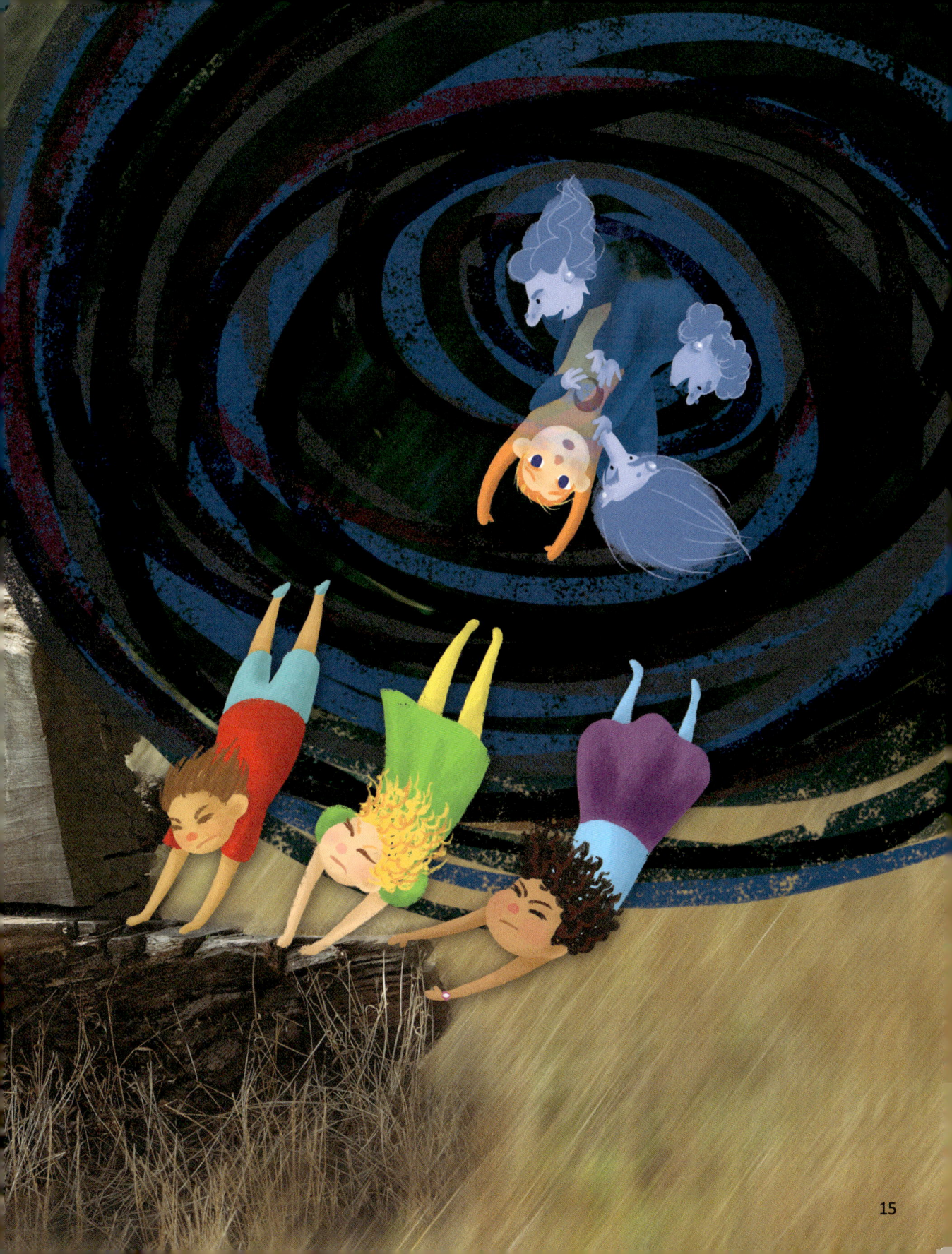

A friendly voice from behind them said "you can save your sister and the world if you listen to me."
To their surprise, there was a platypus! An egg-laying, duck-billed, beaver-tailed, otter-footed mammal that usually lived in Australia. What was this strange animal doing in their park? And could it really help them?
To find out you need to *take another mouthful!*

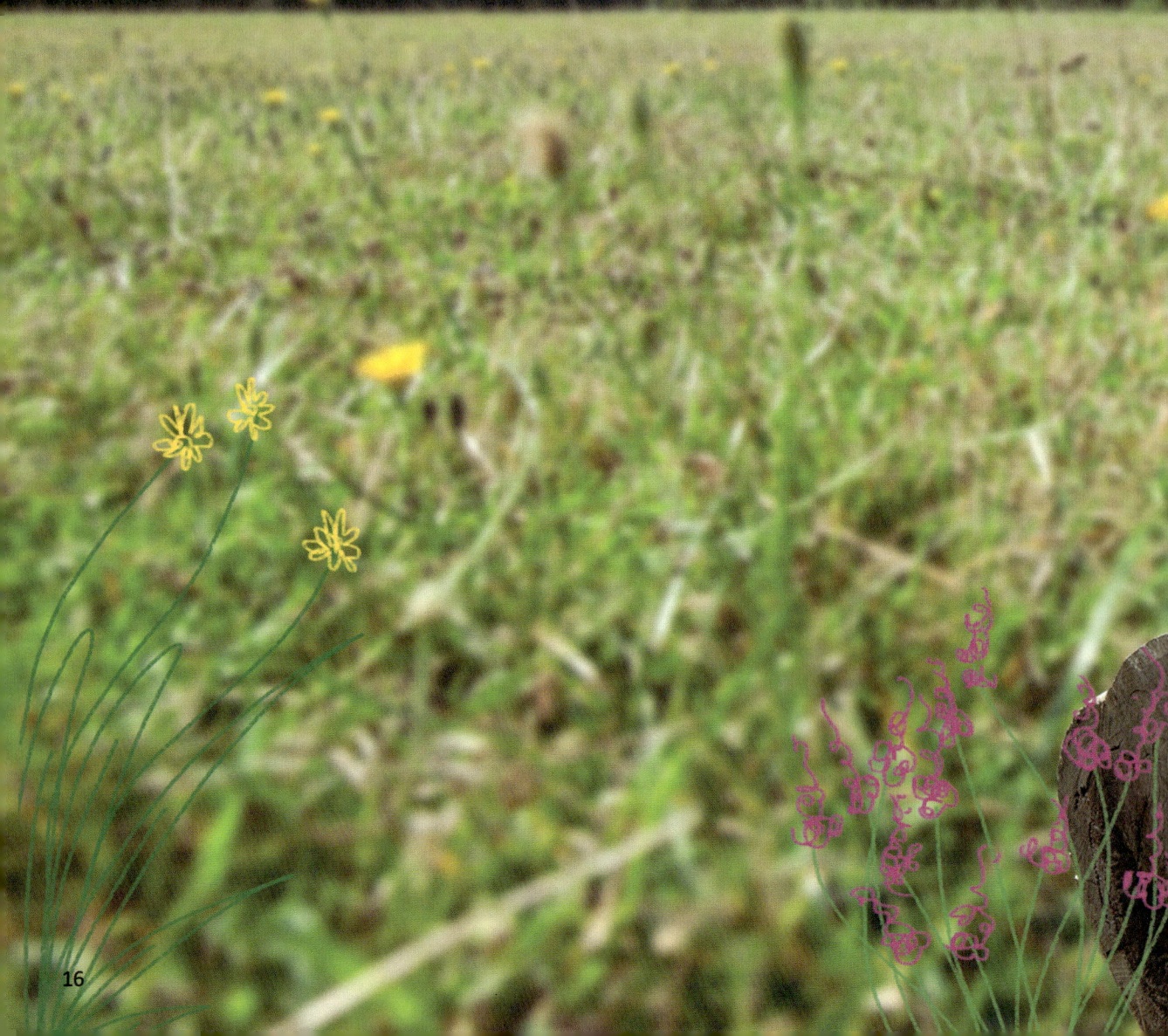

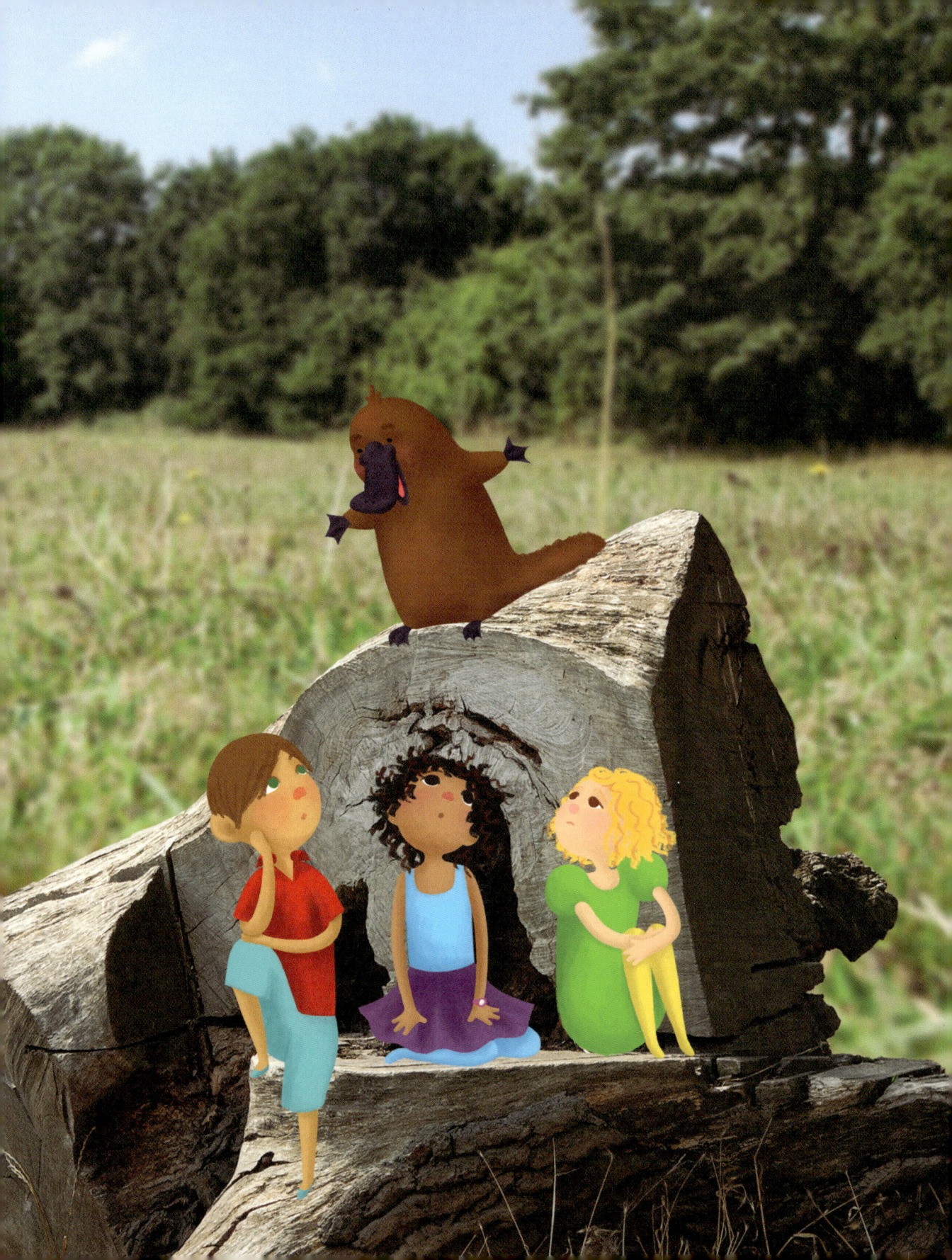

Mr Platypus explained that he was a magical messenger and had been sent by some good witches who lived by the sea. The tornado was in fact magic and had been sent by the greedy, lazy and wicked witches of the sky to gobble up happy children! Their plan was to capture all the children in the world and have them clean their disgusting dirty dishes. To protect yourself and the adventurers, you need to *take another mouthful!*

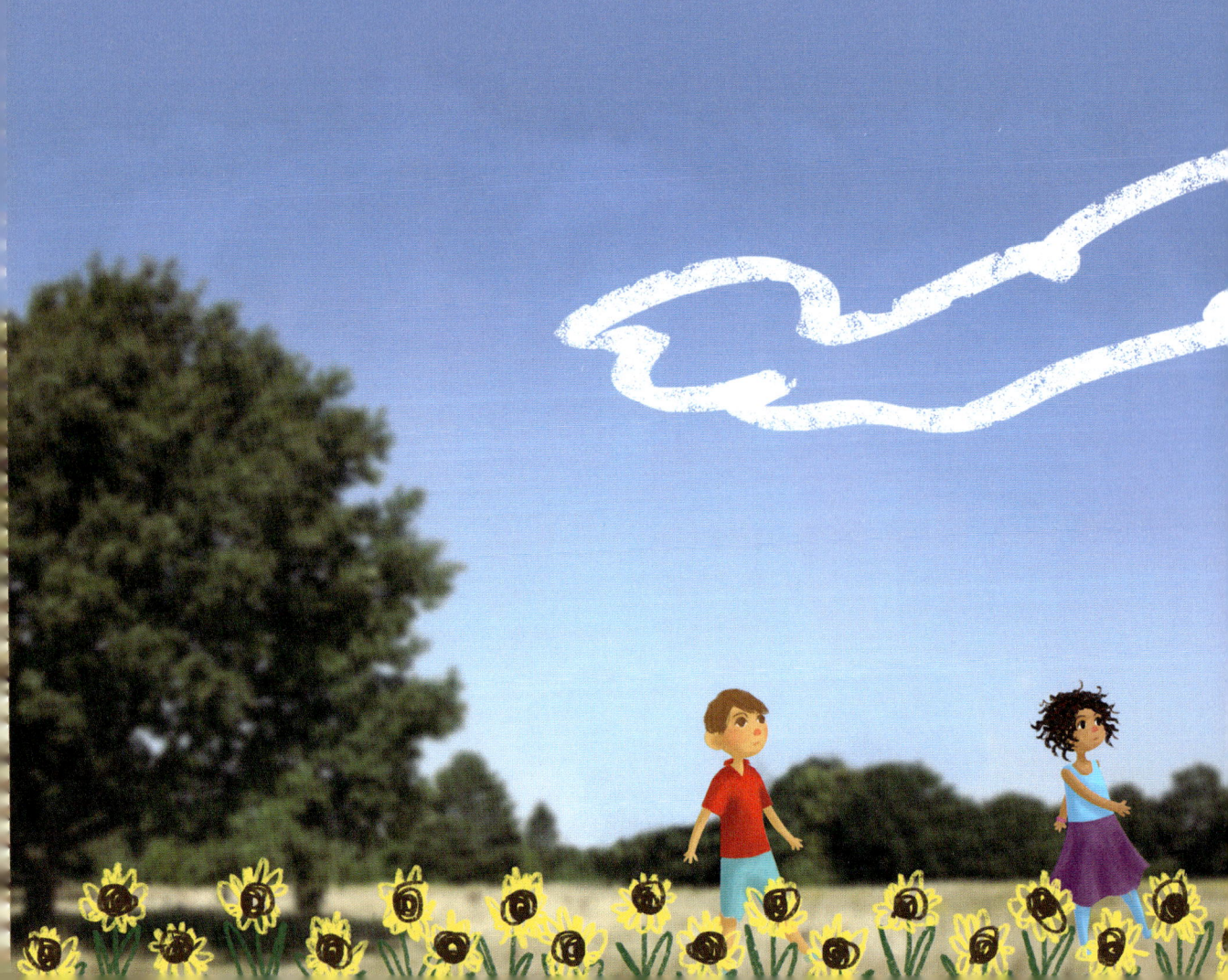

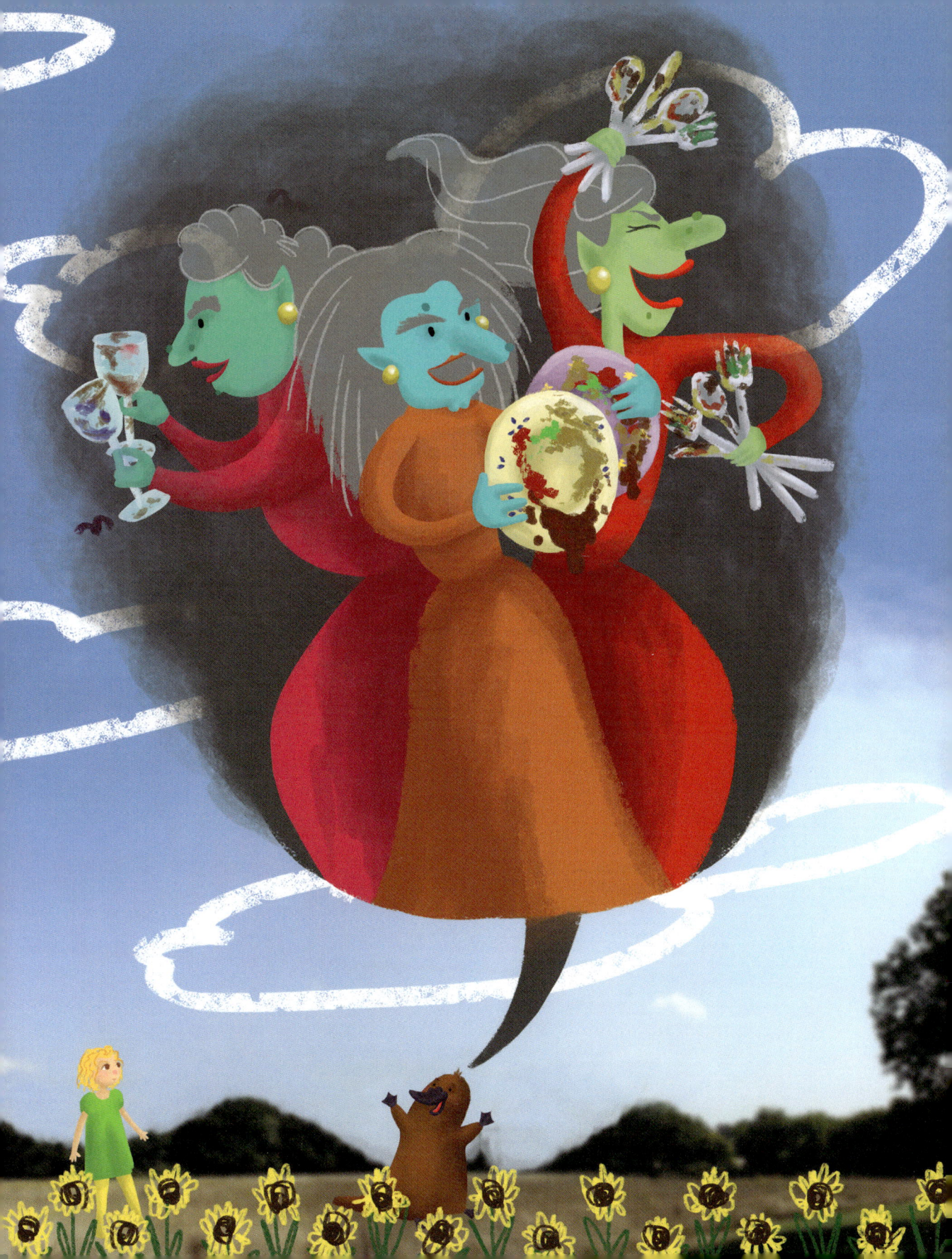

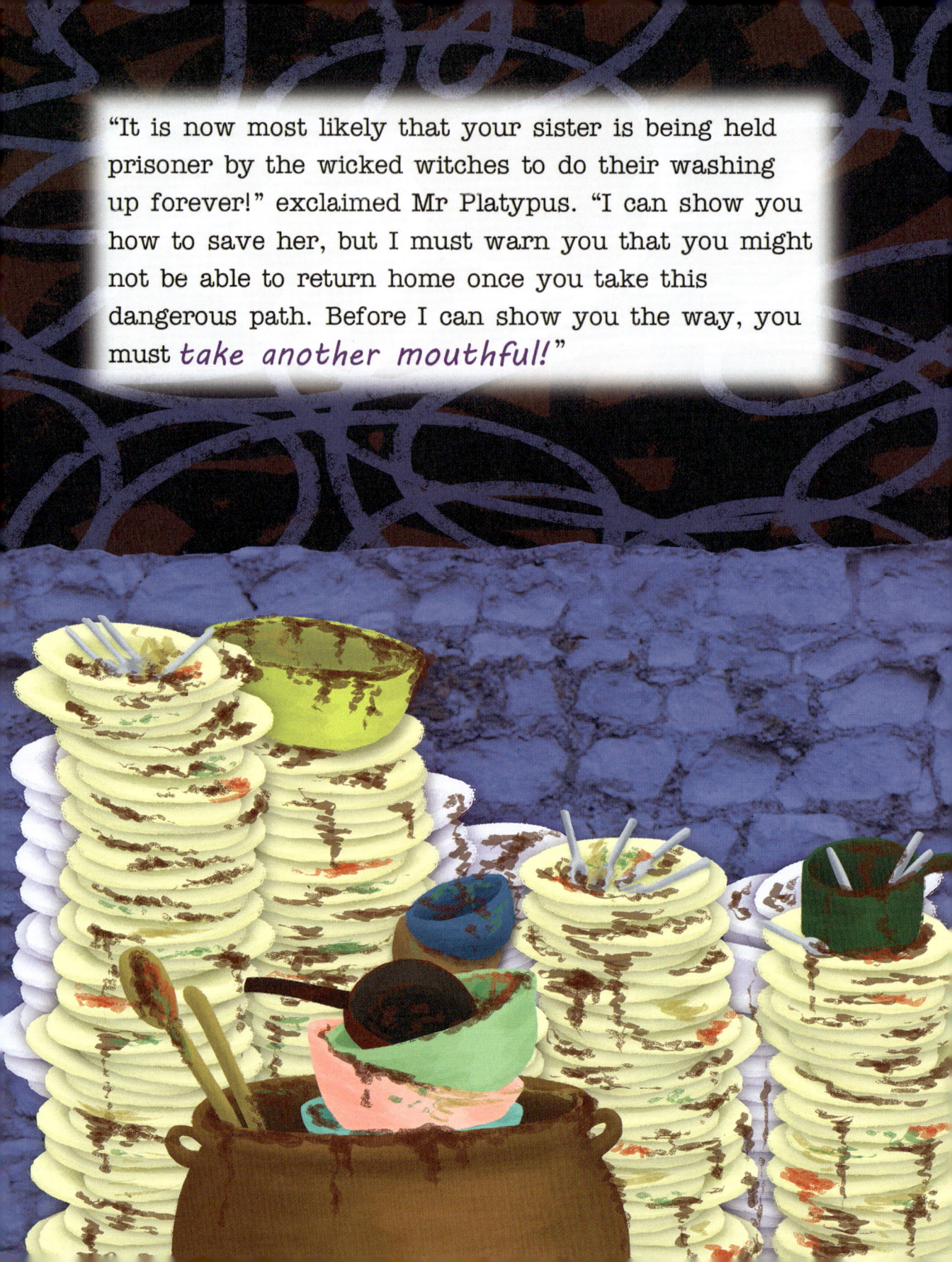

"It is now most likely that your sister is being held prisoner by the wicked witches to do their washing up forever!" exclaimed Mr Platypus. "I can show you how to save her, but I must warn you that you might not be able to return home once you take this dangerous path. Before I can show you the way, you must *take another mouthful!*"

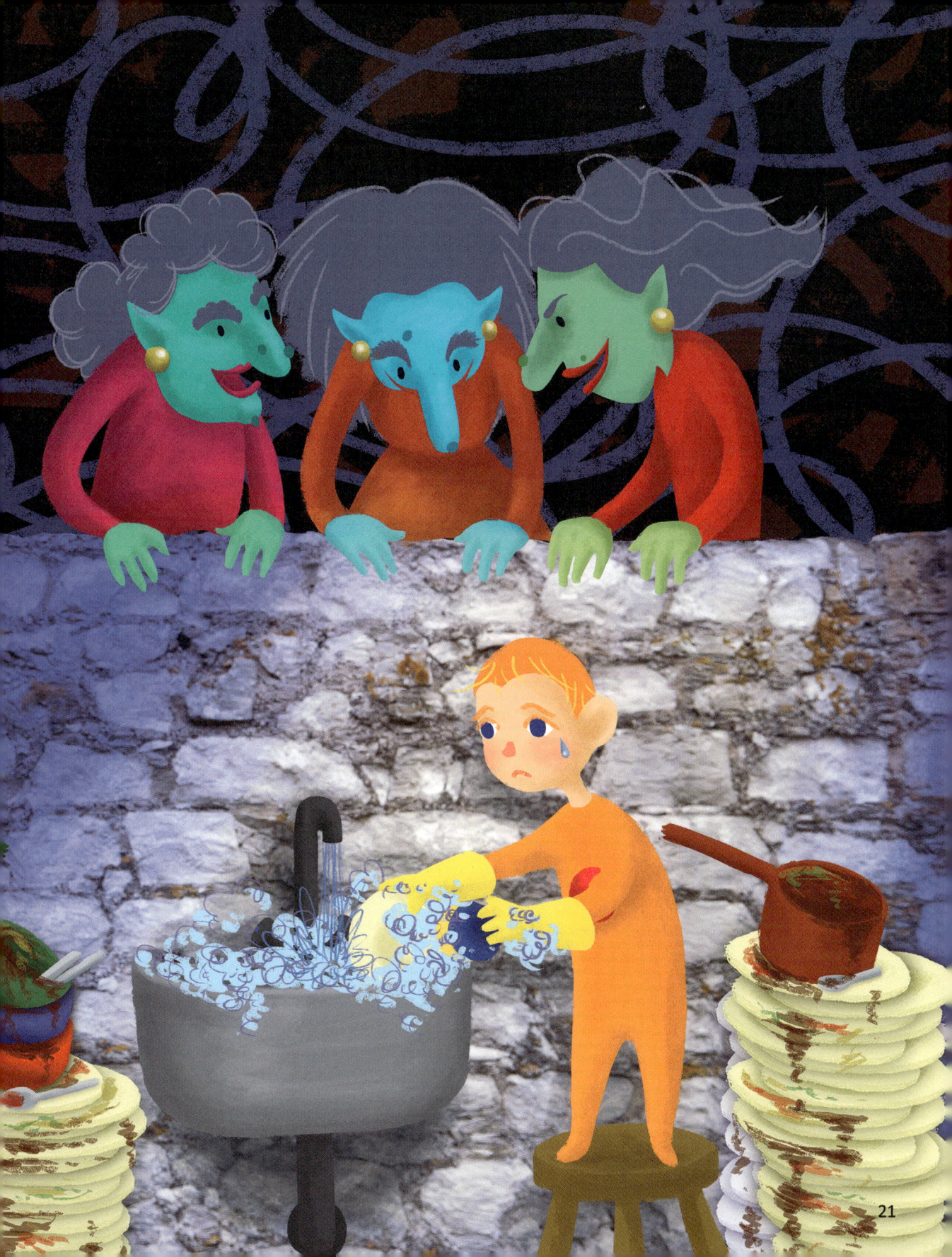

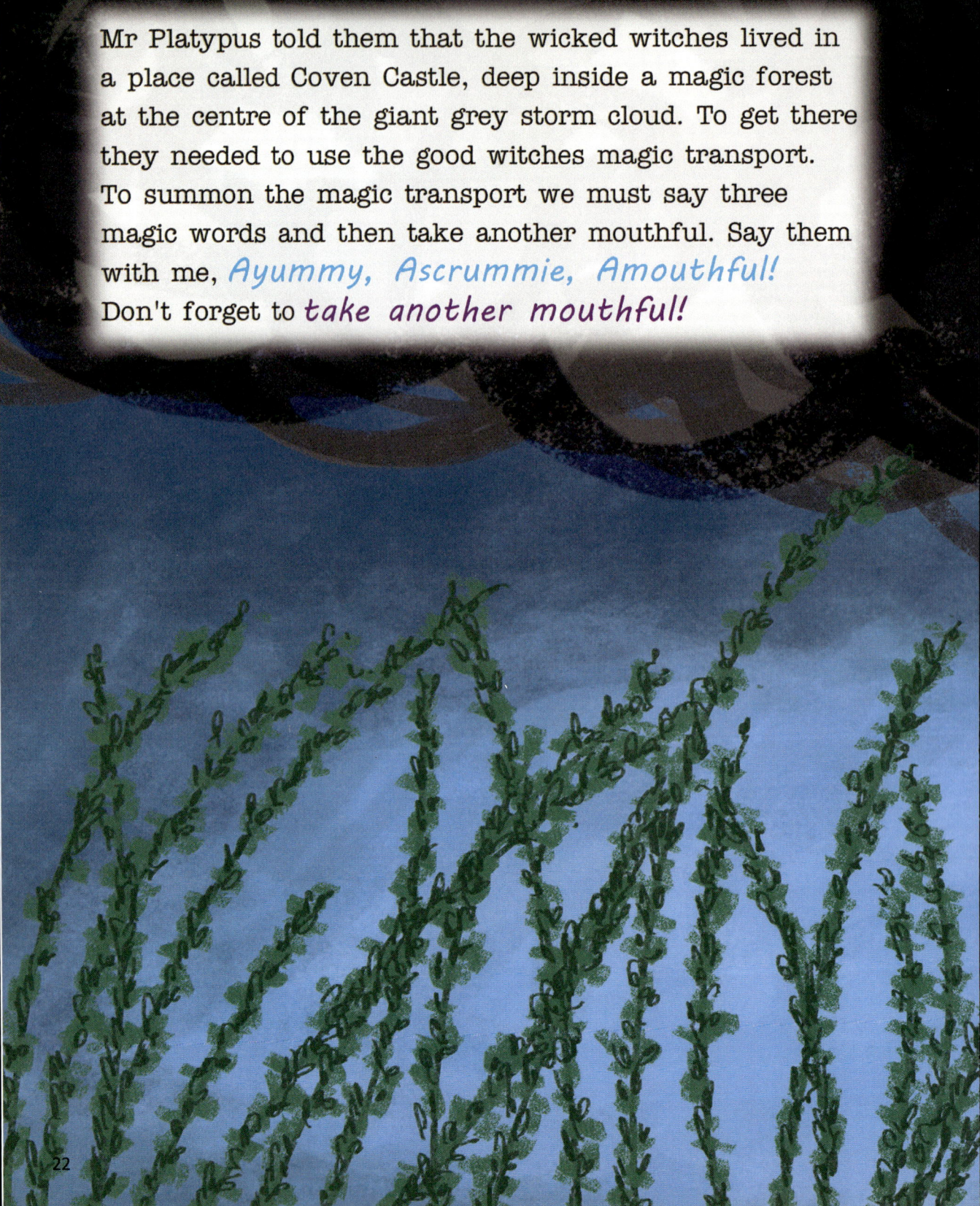

Mr Platypus told them that the wicked witches lived in a place called Coven Castle, deep inside a magic forest at the centre of the giant grey storm cloud. To get there they needed to use the good witches magic transport. To summon the magic transport we must say three magic words and then take another mouthful. Say them with me, *Ayummy, Ascrummie, Amouthful!* Don't forget to *take another mouthful!*

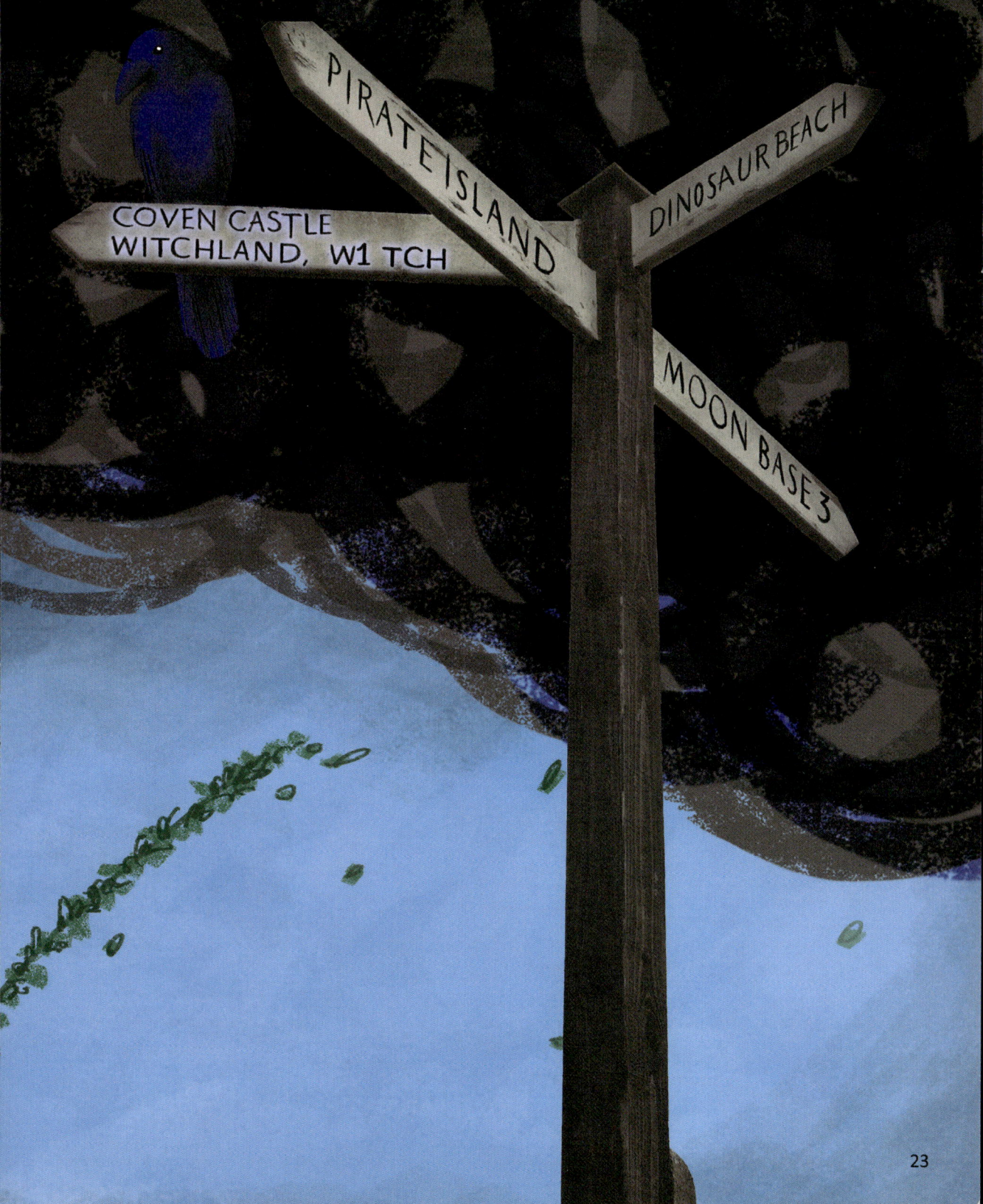

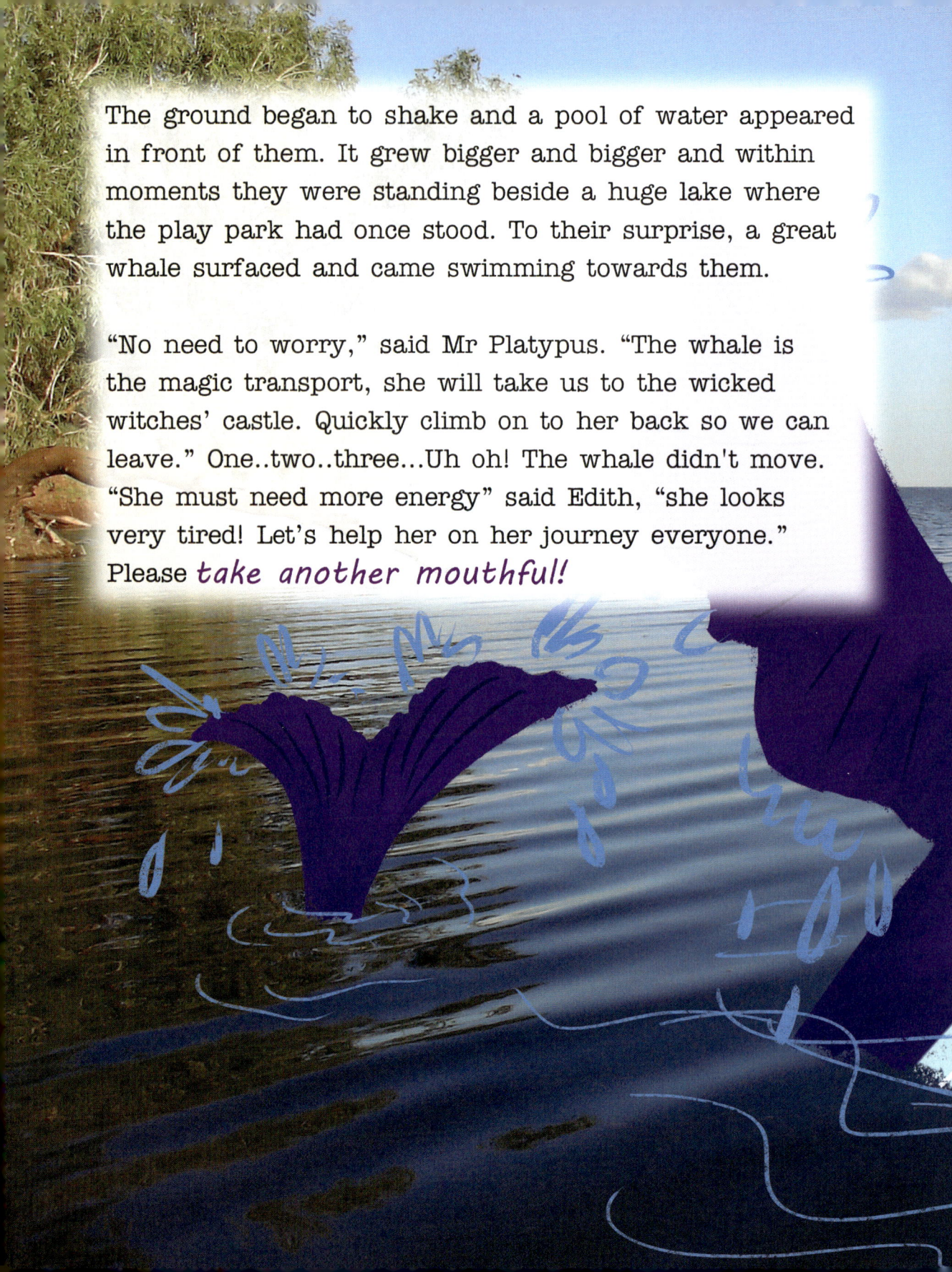

The ground began to shake and a pool of water appeared in front of them. It grew bigger and bigger and within moments they were standing beside a huge lake where the play park had once stood. To their surprise, a great whale surfaced and came swimming towards them.

"No need to worry," said Mr Platypus. "The whale is the magic transport, she will take us to the wicked witches' castle. Quickly climb on to her back so we can leave." One..two..three...Uh oh! The whale didn't move. "She must need more energy" said Edith, "she looks very tired! Let's help her on her journey everyone." Please *take another mouthful!*

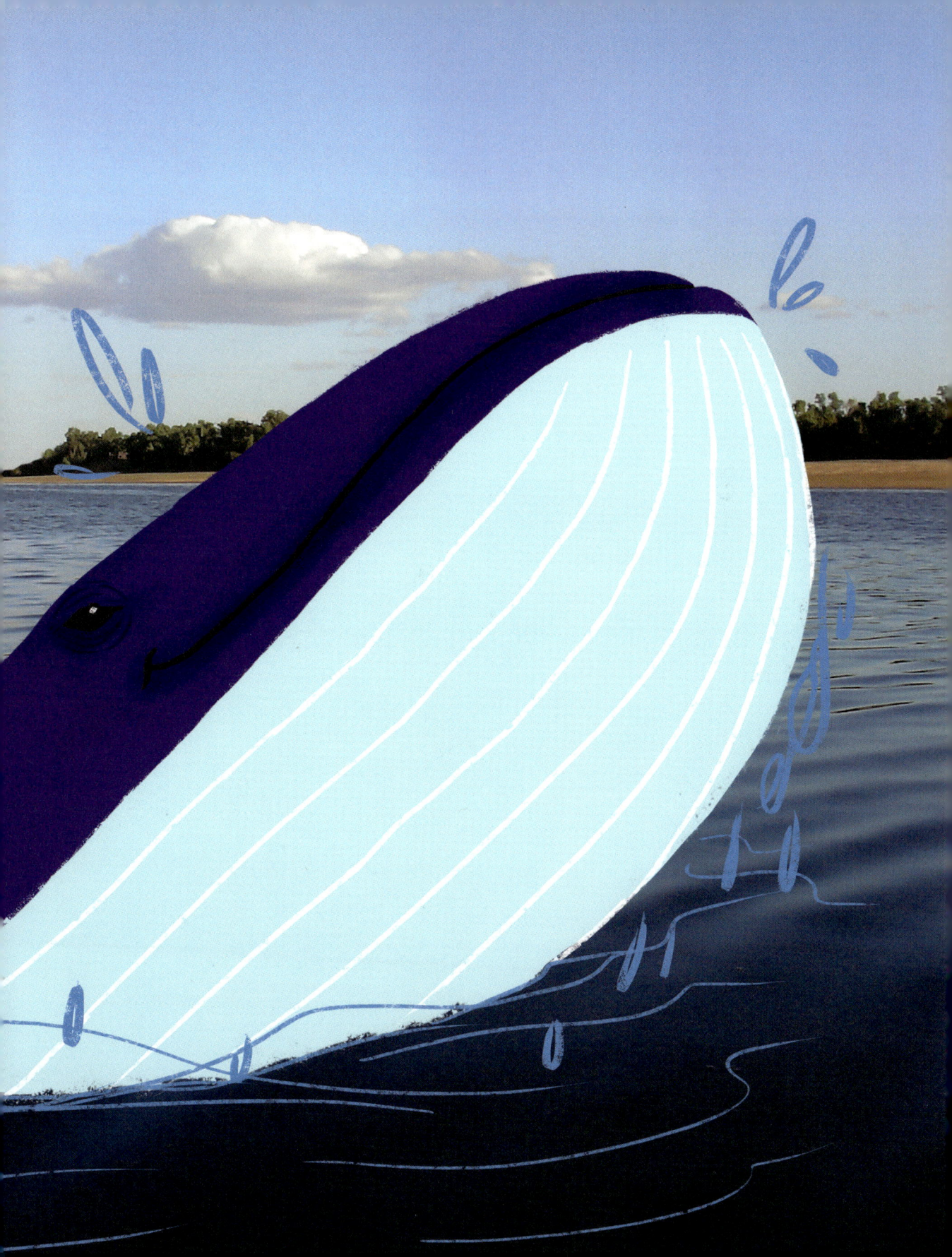

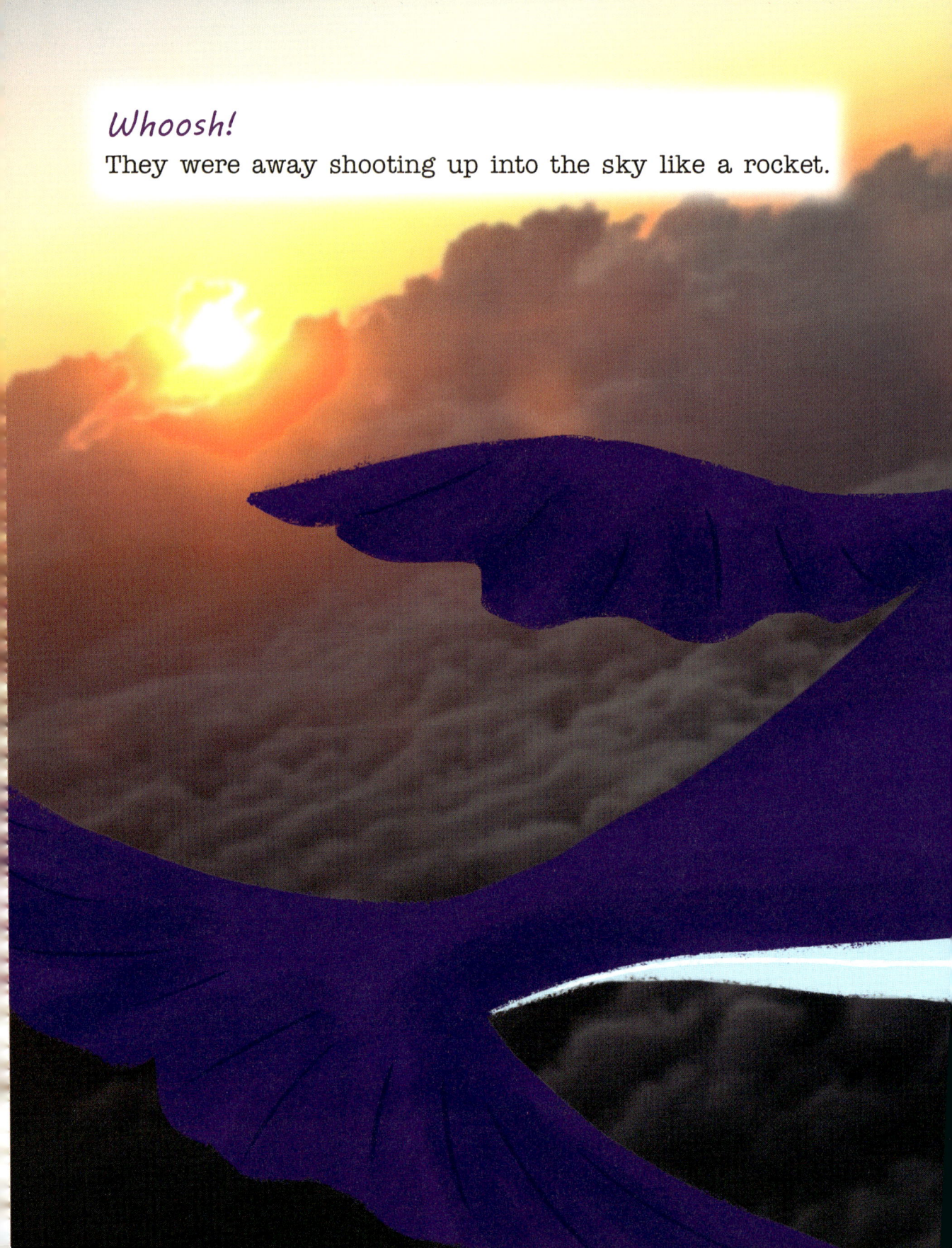

Whoosh!
They were away shooting up into the sky like a rocket.

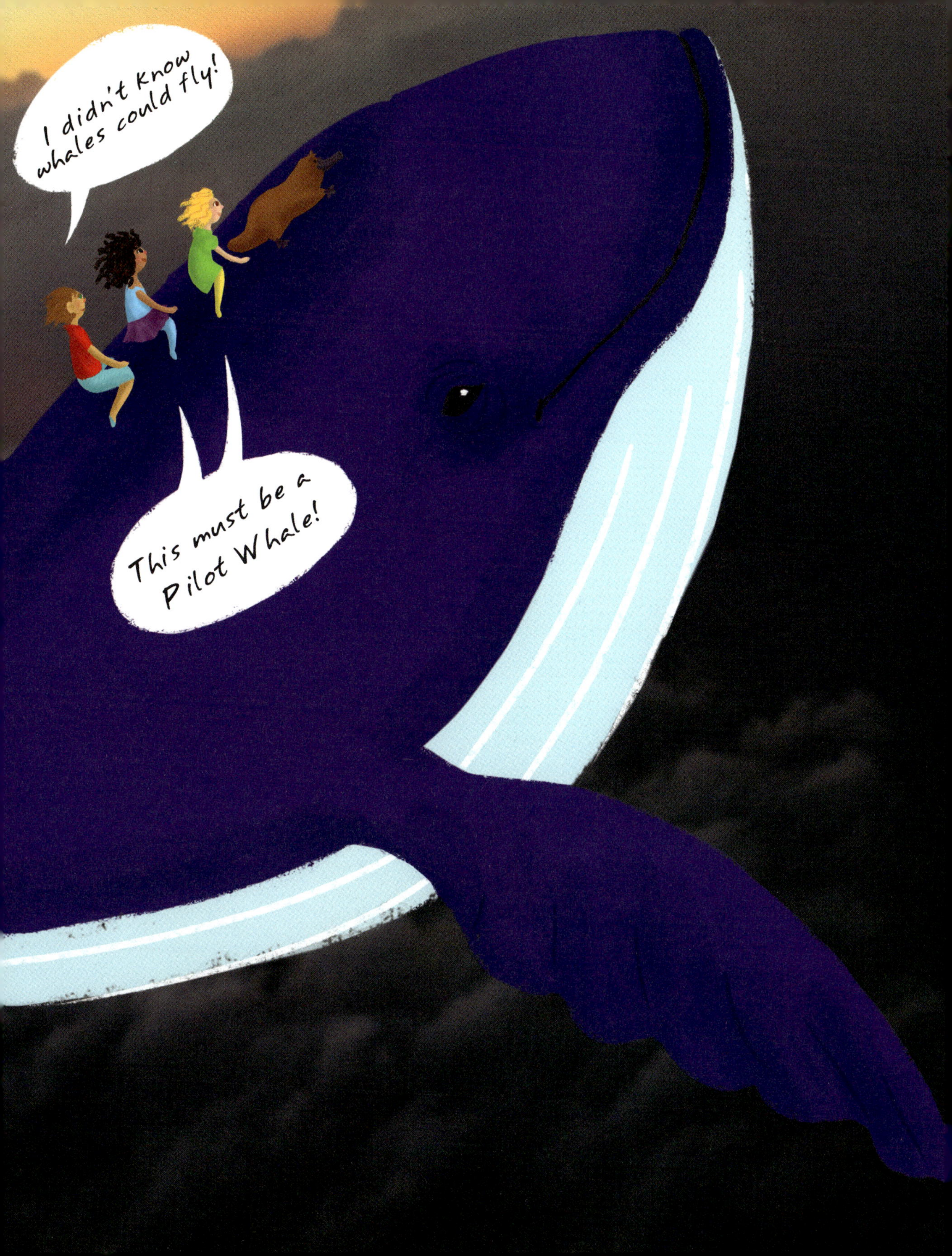
I didn't know whales could fly!
This must be a Pilot Whale!

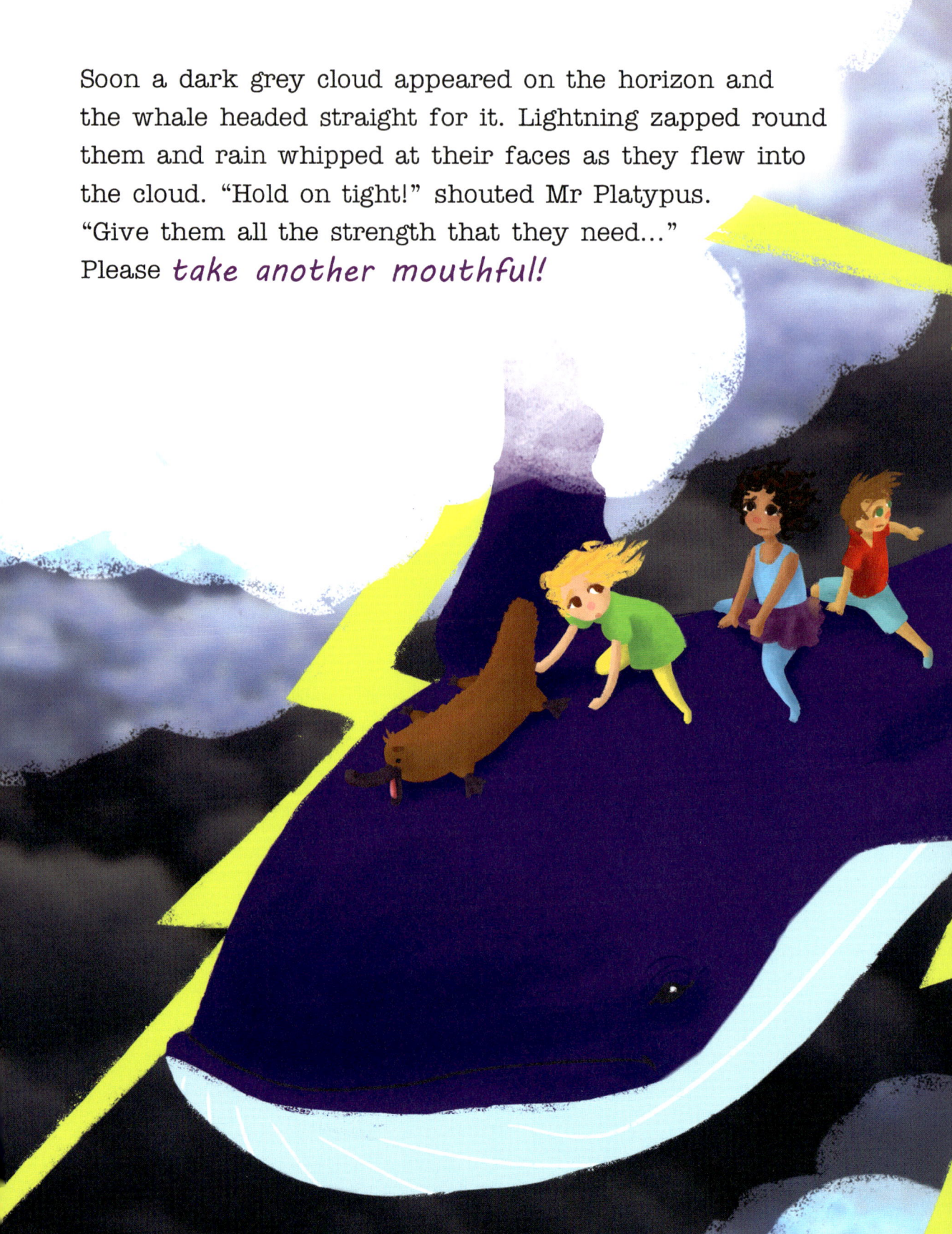

Soon a dark grey cloud appeared on the horizon and the whale headed straight for it. Lightning zapped round them and rain whipped at their faces as they flew into the cloud. "Hold on tight!" shouted Mr Platypus. "Give them all the strength that they need..."
Please *take another mouthful!*

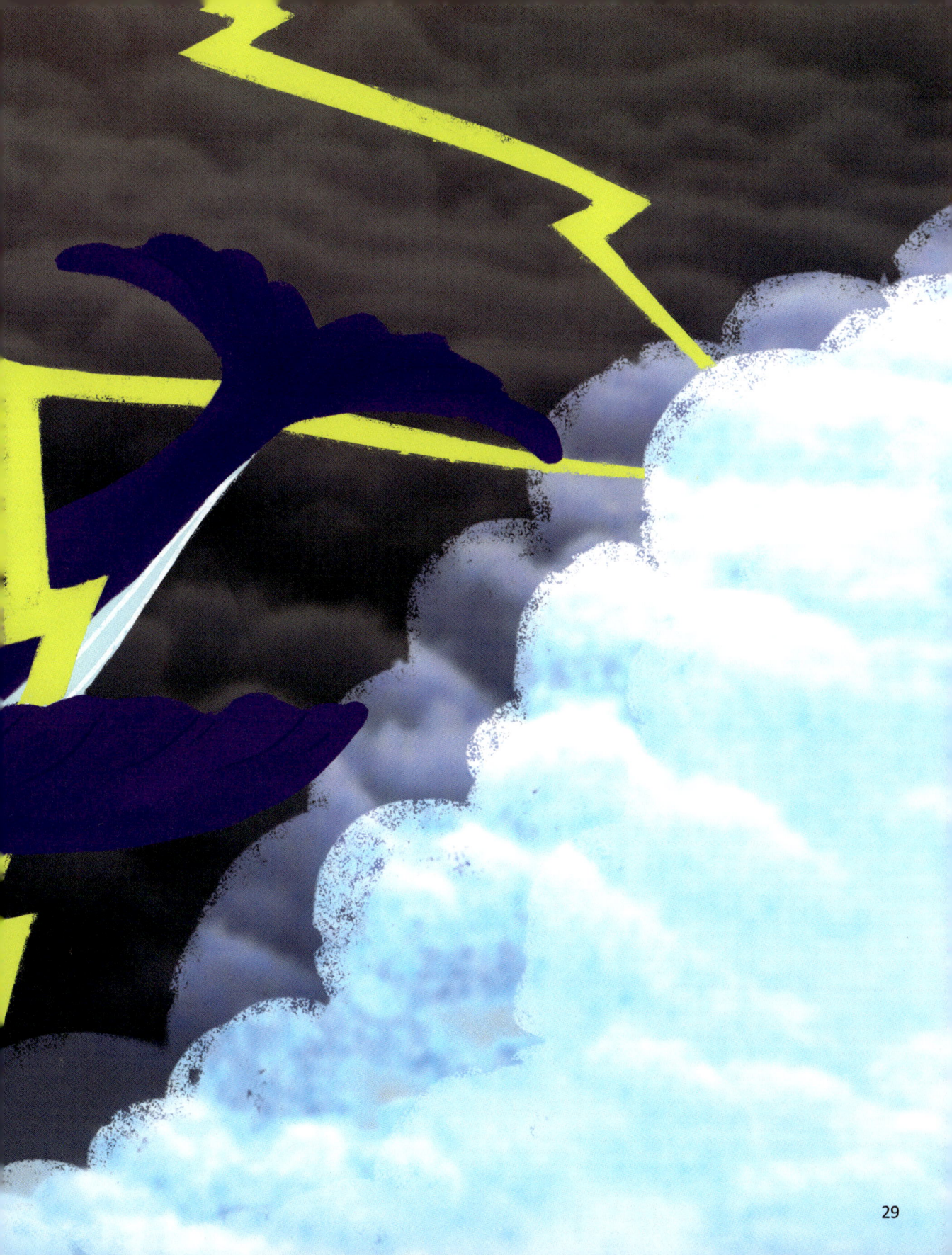

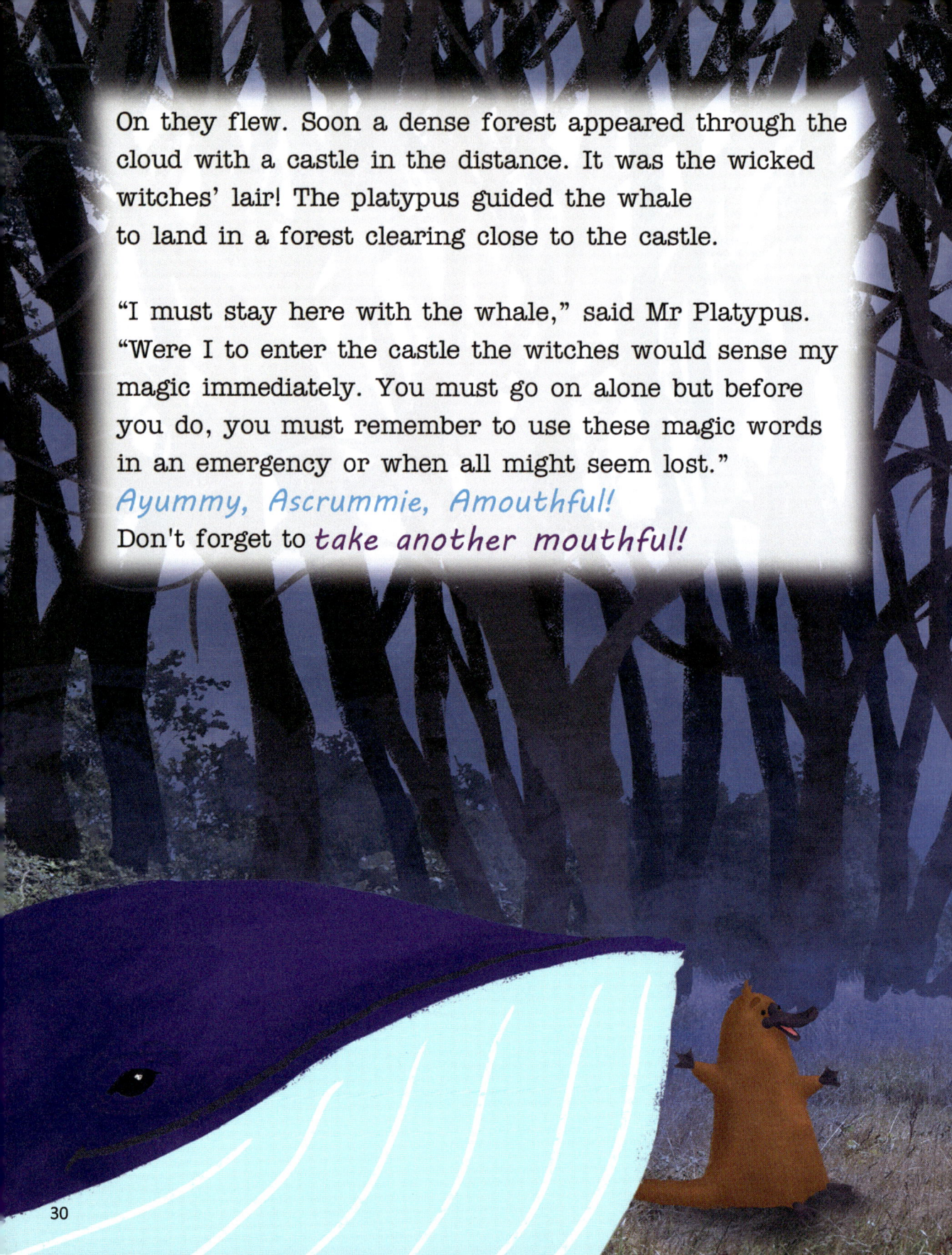

On they flew. Soon a dense forest appeared through the cloud with a castle in the distance. It was the wicked witches' lair! The platypus guided the whale to land in a forest clearing close to the castle.

"I must stay here with the whale," said Mr Platypus. "Were I to enter the castle the witches would sense my magic immediately. You must go on alone but before you do, you must remember to use these magic words in an emergency or when all might seem lost."
Ayummy, Ascrummie, Amouthful!
Don't forget to *take another mouthful!*

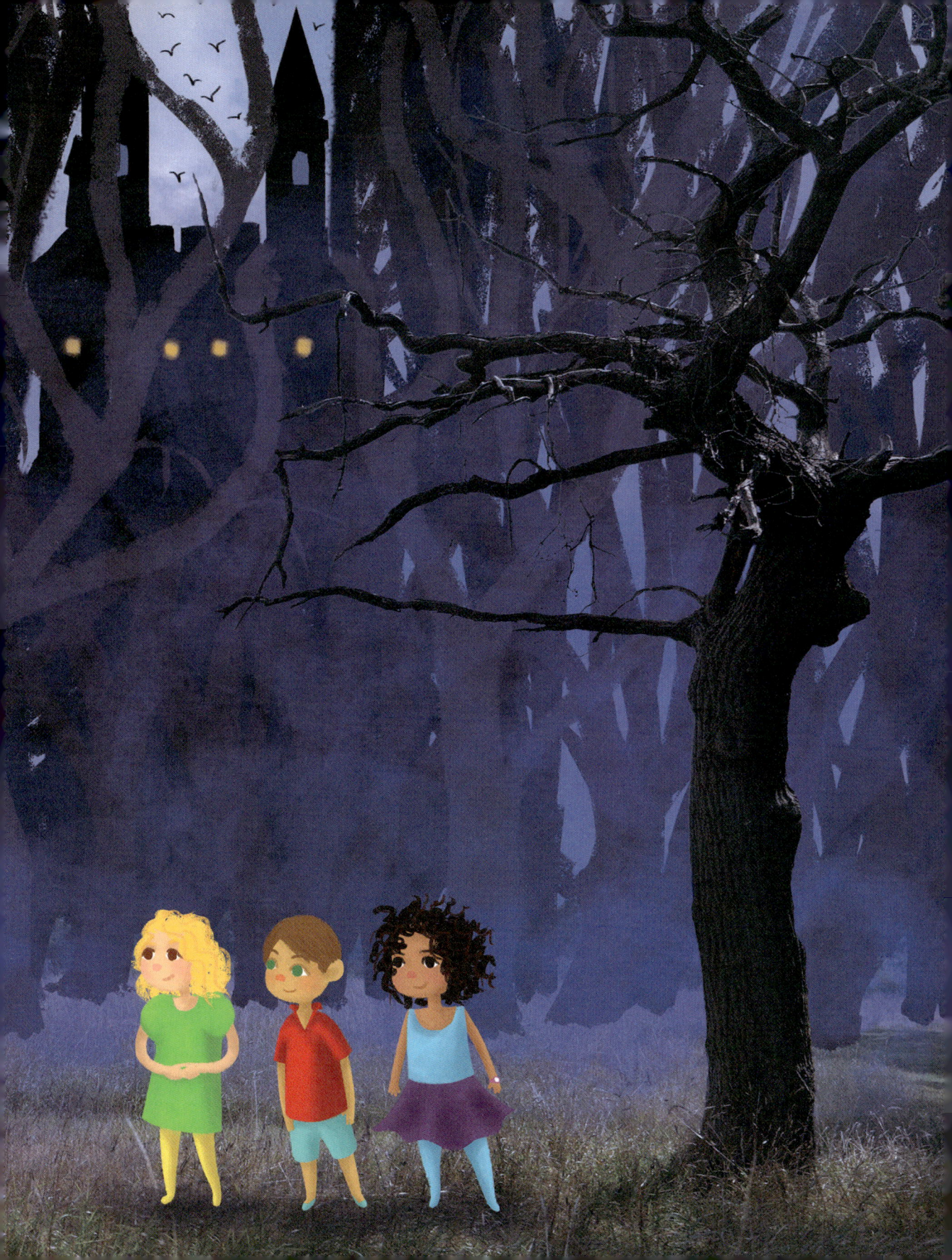

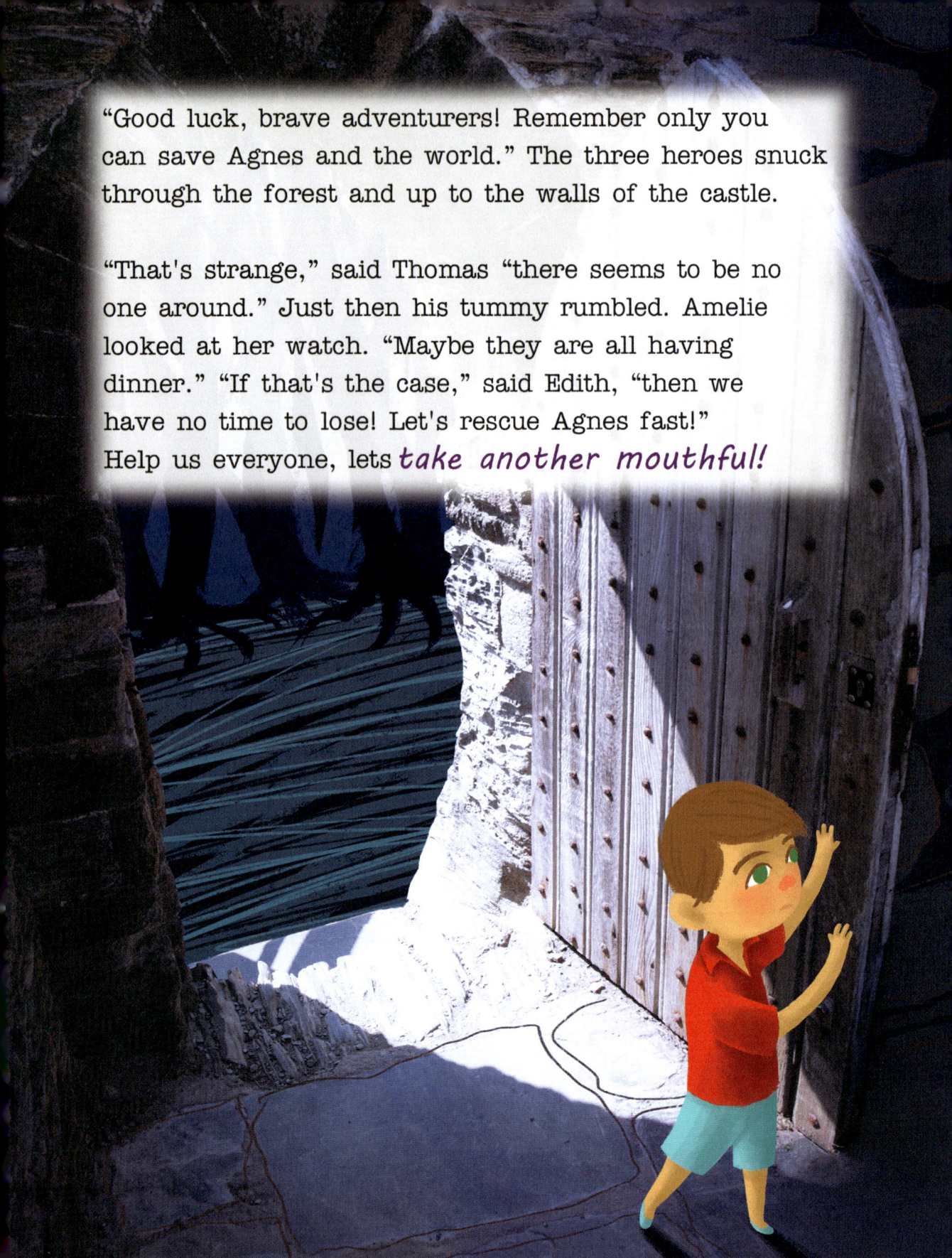

"Good luck, brave adventurers! Remember only you can save Agnes and the world." The three heroes snuck through the forest and up to the walls of the castle.

"That's strange," said Thomas "there seems to be no one around." Just then his tummy rumbled. Amelie looked at her watch. "Maybe they are all having dinner." "If that's the case," said Edith, "then we have no time to lose! Let's rescue Agnes fast!" Help us everyone, lets *take another mouthful!*

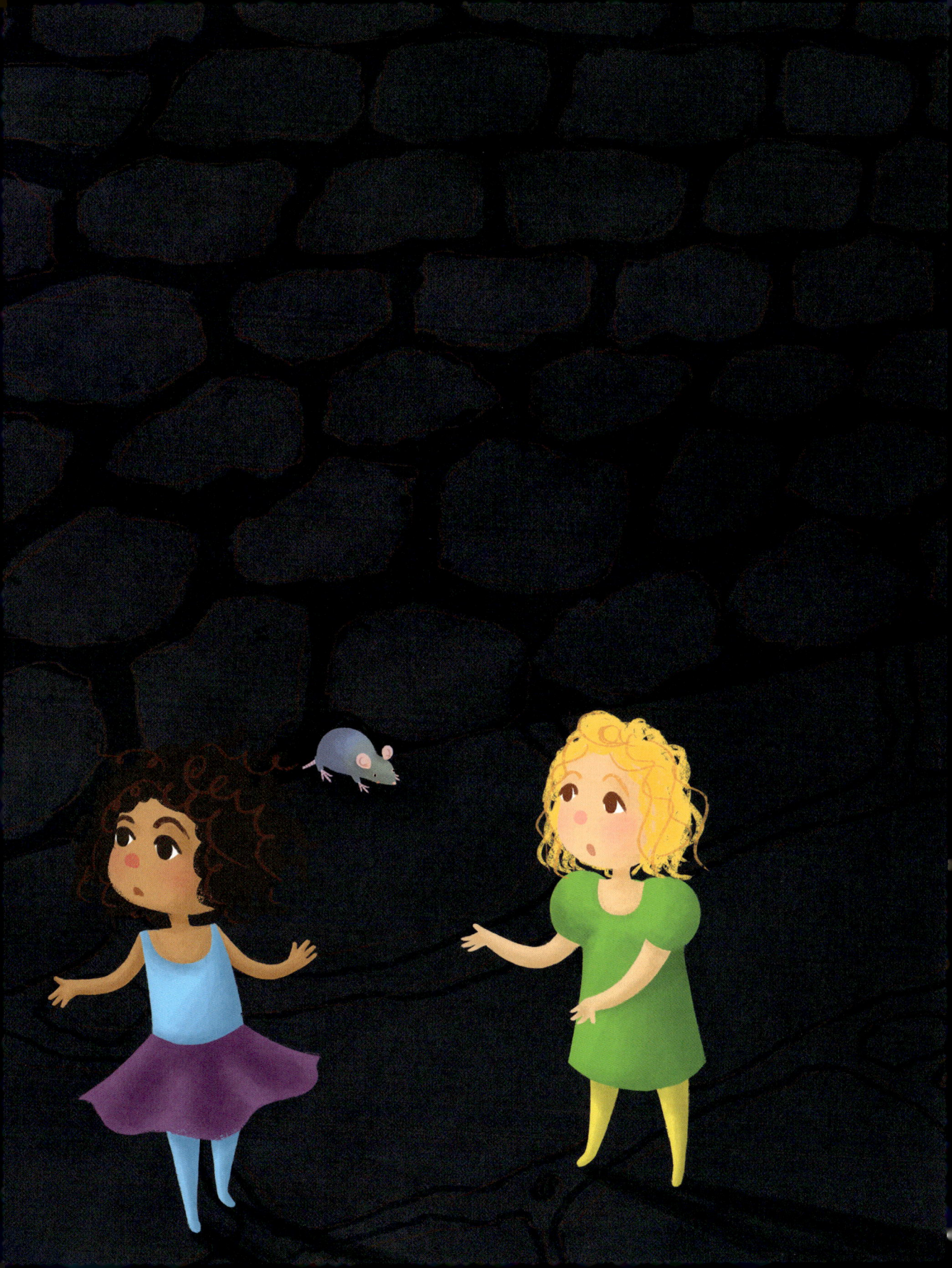

As they entered the castle they heard the sound of crockery clinking and cutlery clanking. They followed the sound and came to a great hall and found it full of witches!

There were: Tall witches, short witches, green witches, blue witches, witches covered in warts and witches covered in sauce! And all of them munching and crunching and chewing and slurping down their dinner. Make sure they don't spot you and quick, *take another mouthful!*

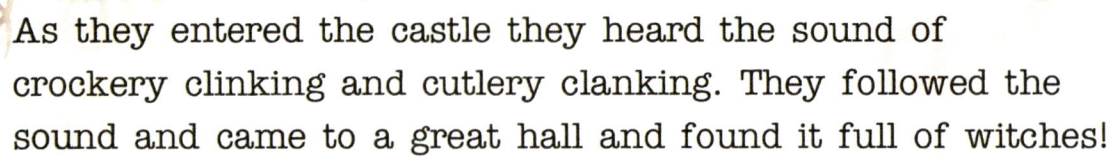

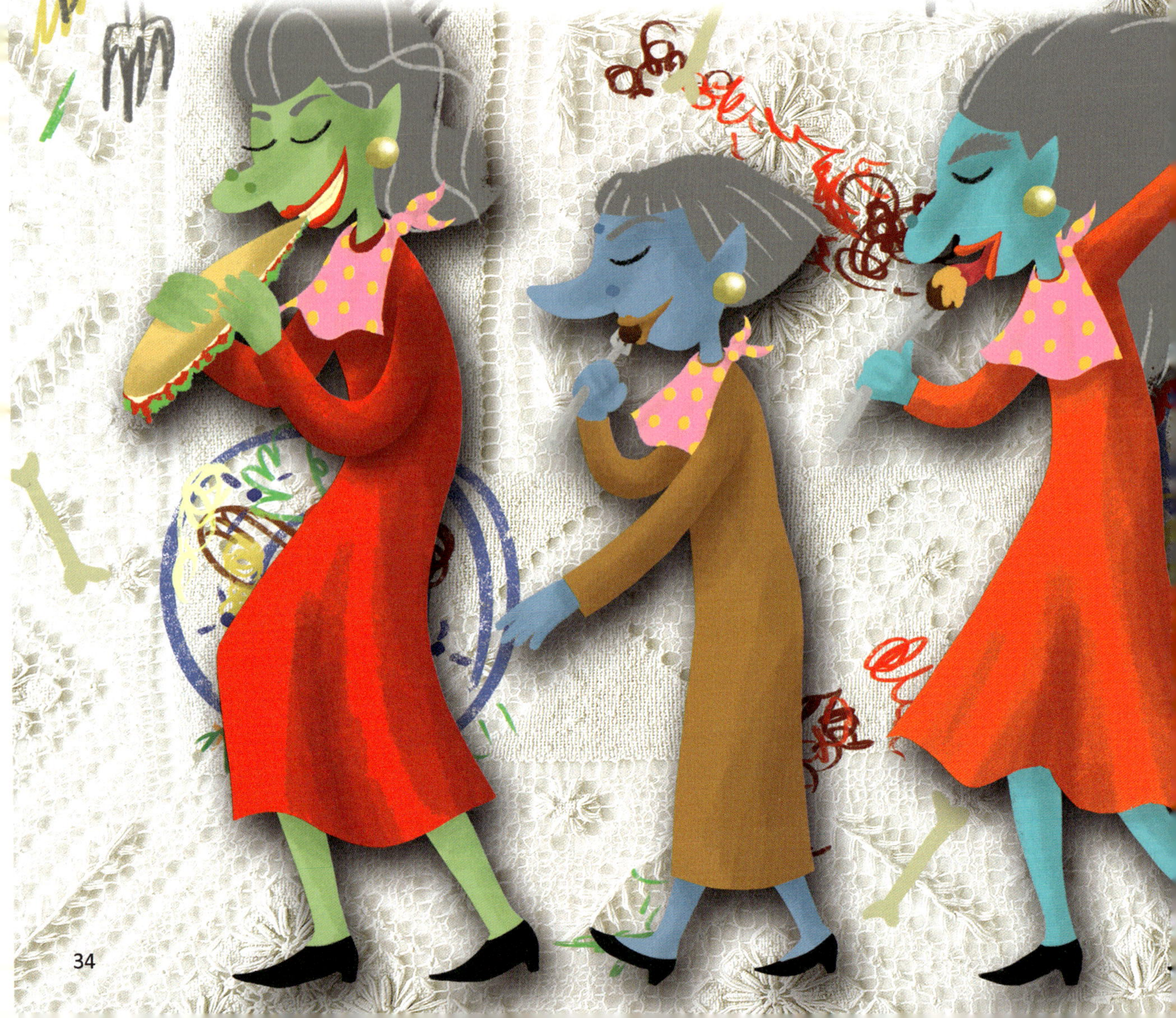

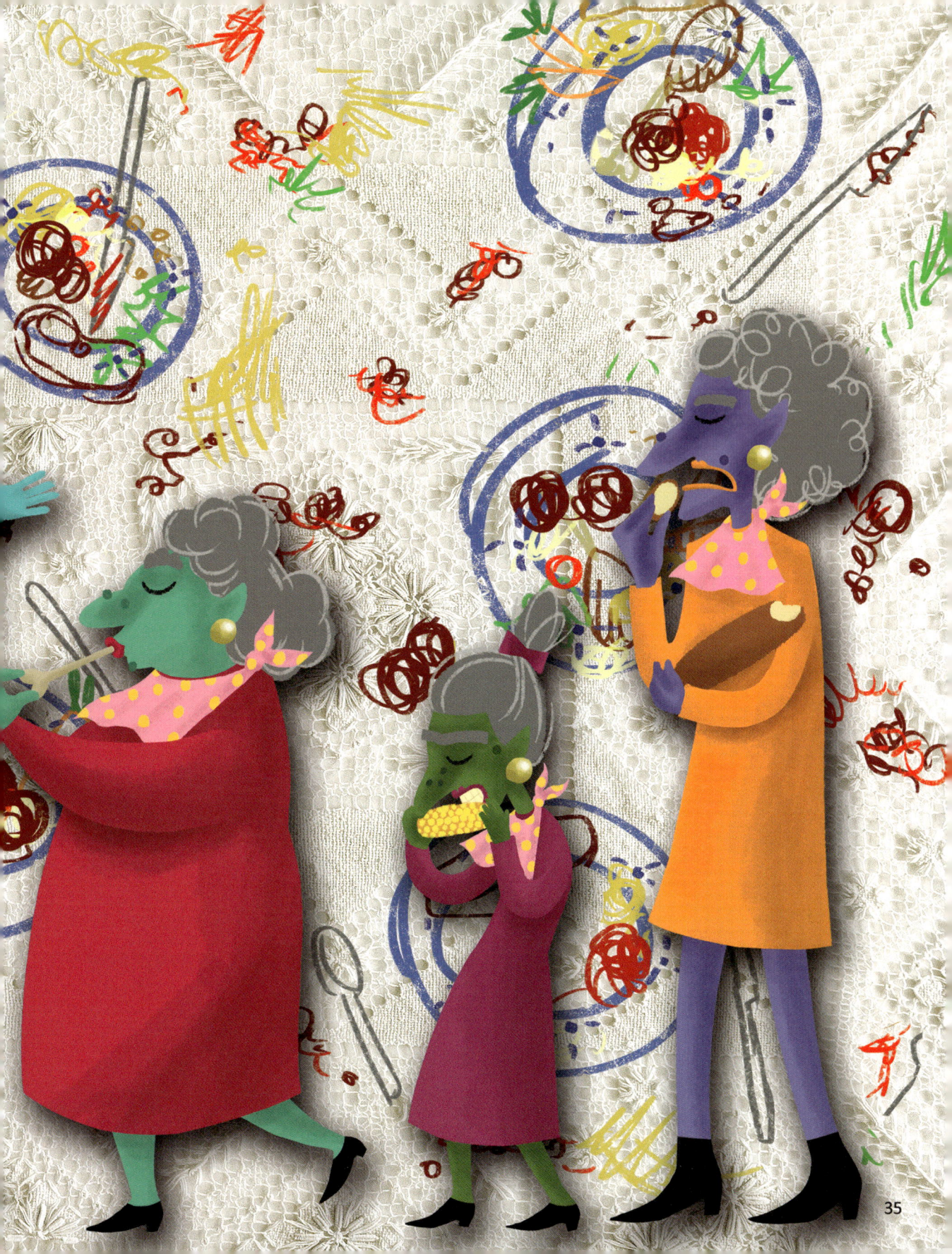

The adventurers were searching for the kitchen. As they tiptoed down a small dark passage to the side of the hall they walked straight into a door.

"It's locked!" gasped Thomas as he tried the handle. There was some old writing carved into the door. The chidren read:

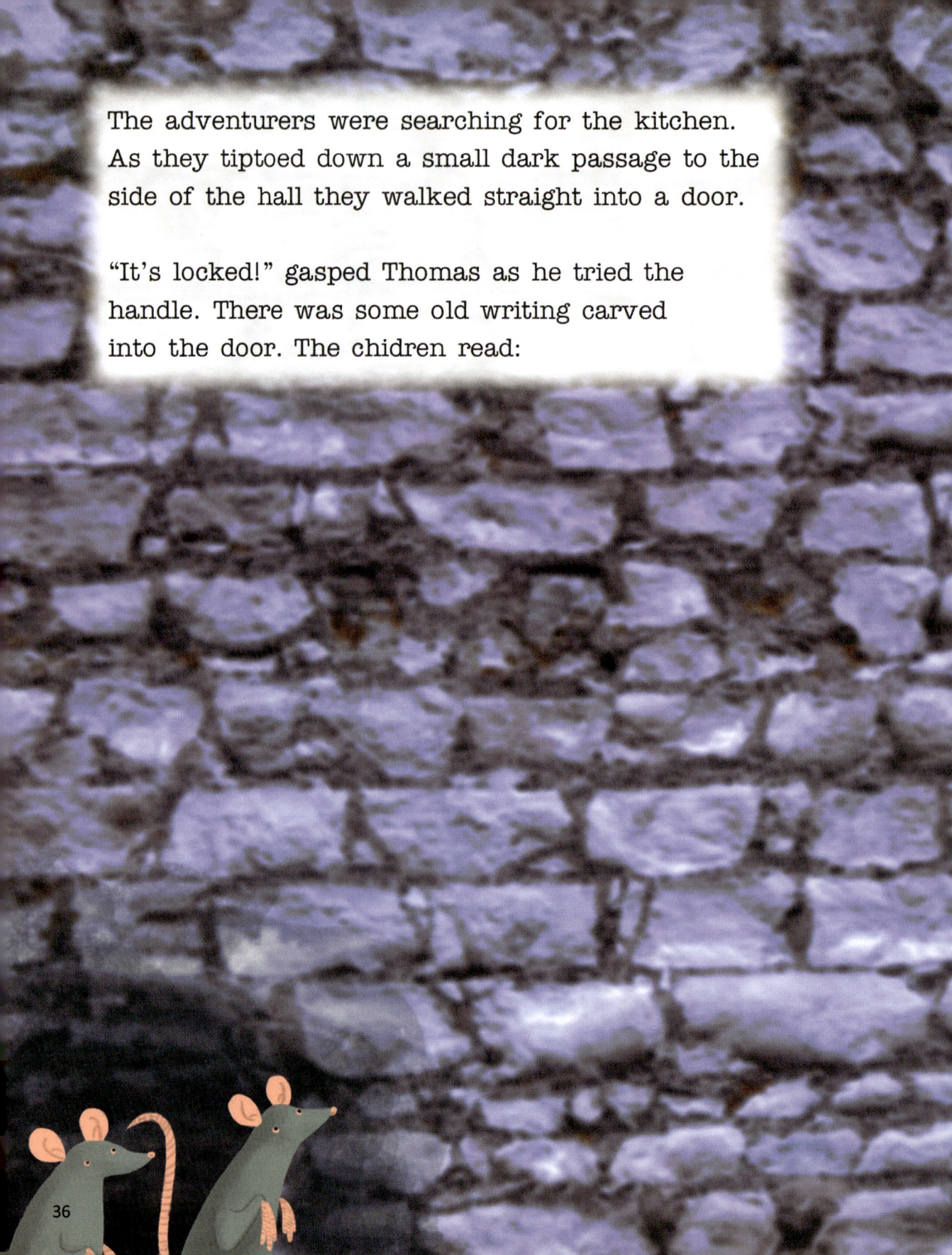

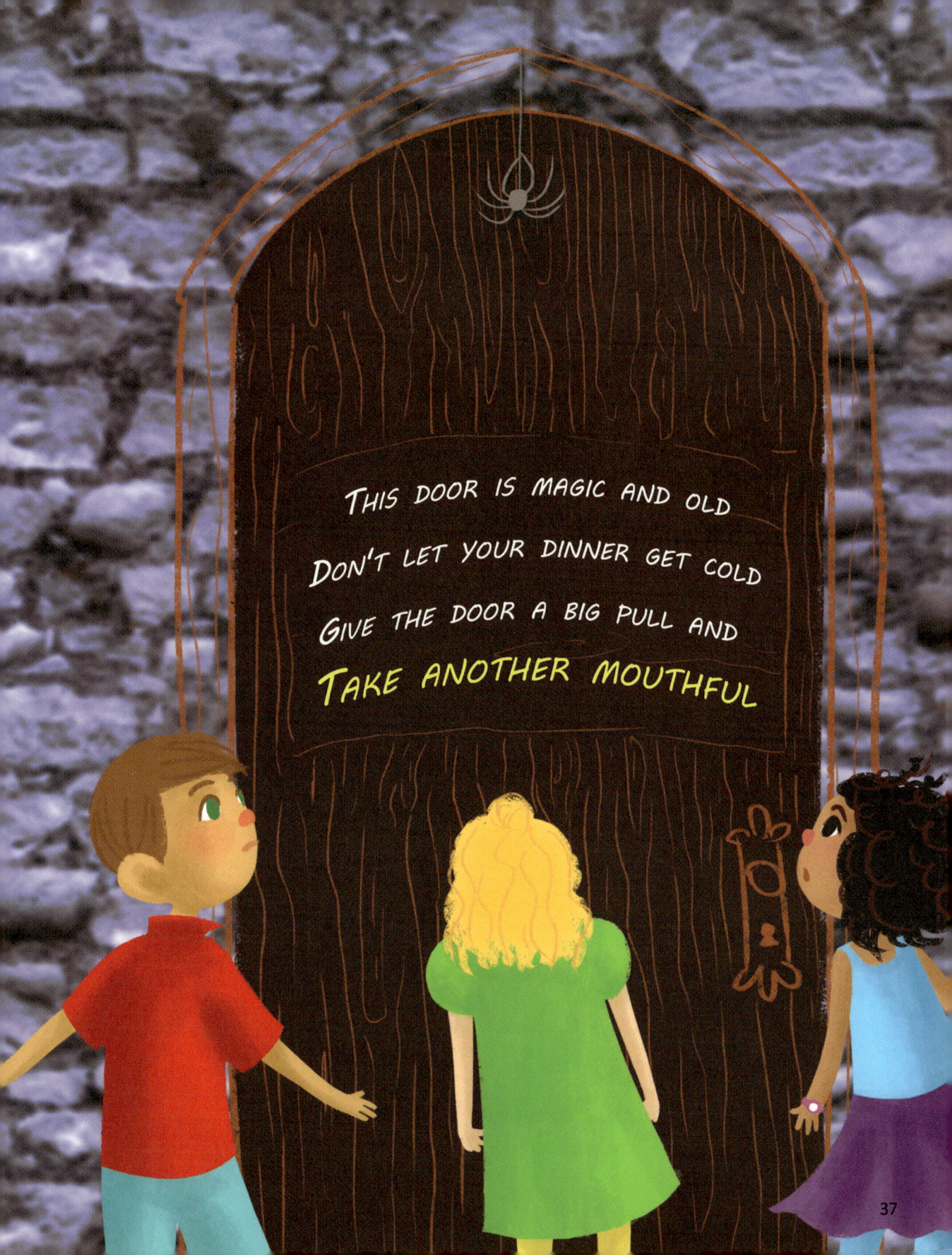

This door is magic and old
Don't let your dinner get cold
Give the door a big pull and
Take another mouthful

The door swung open with a creak. There, stood by a large kitchen sink, surrounded by bubbles and dirty plates... was Agnes. "Thank goodness you found me! I don't mind washing up at home but there are hundreds of witches and they never stop eating!"

As Agnes ran from the sink, her foot knocked a towering pile of plates which began rocking and swaying above them.

The four hurtled back through the kitchen door just as the plates came crashing down behind them! Several witches heard the smash and dashed straight to the kitchen to investigate. Help our heroes escape and *take another mouthful!*

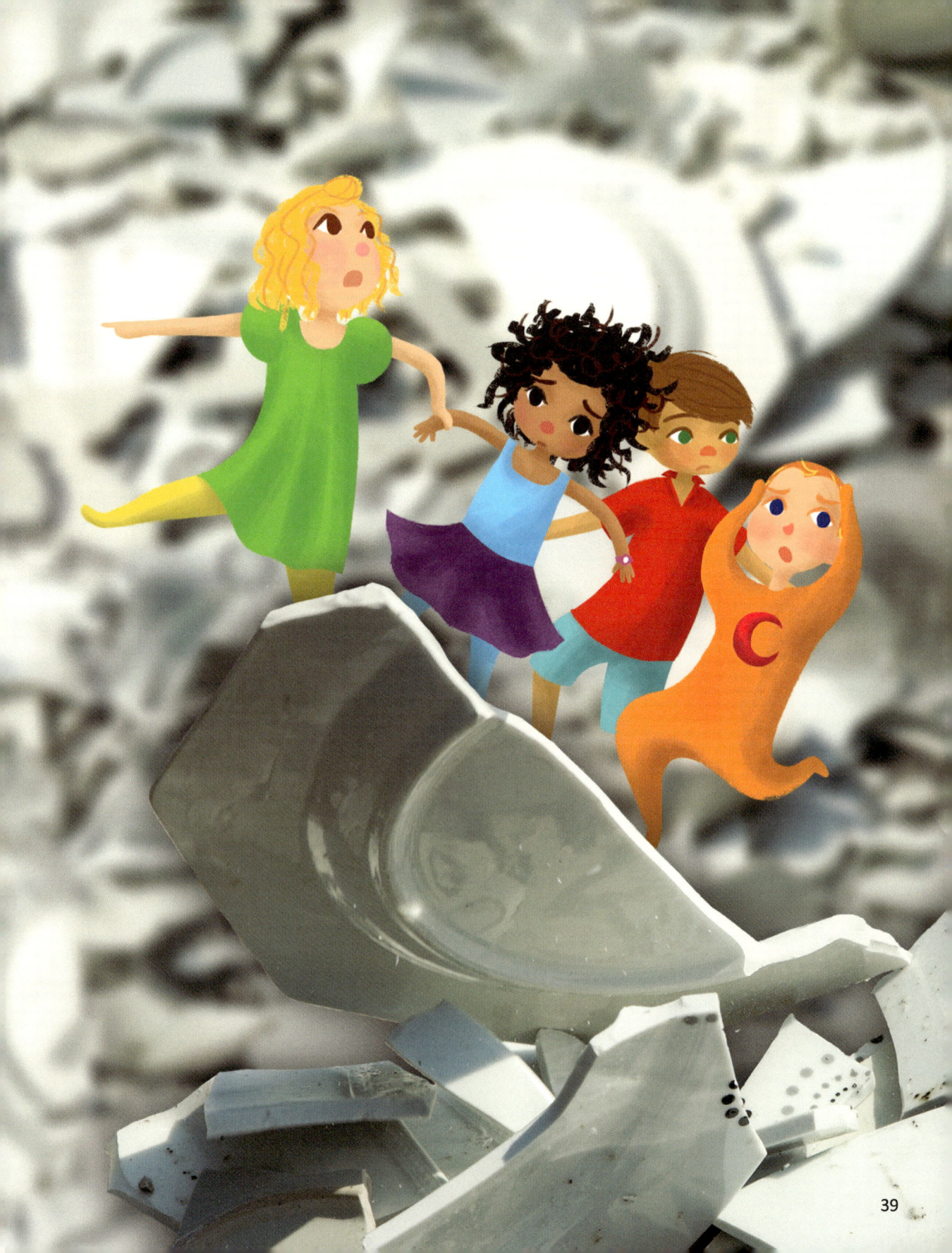

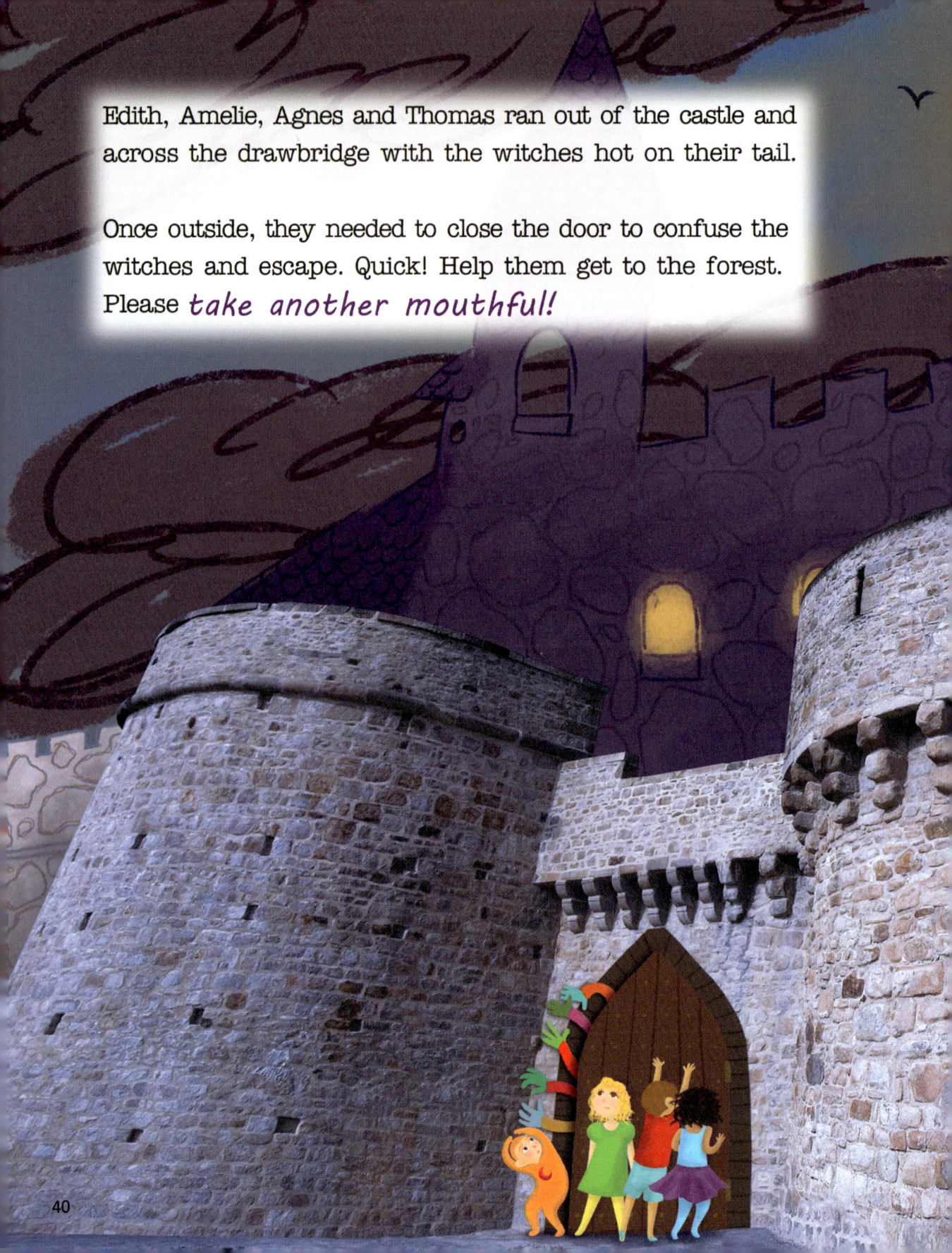

Edith, Amelie, Agnes and Thomas ran out of the castle and across the drawbridge with the witches hot on their tail.

Once outside, they needed to close the door to confuse the witches and escape. Quick! Help them get to the forest. Please *take another mouthful!*

41

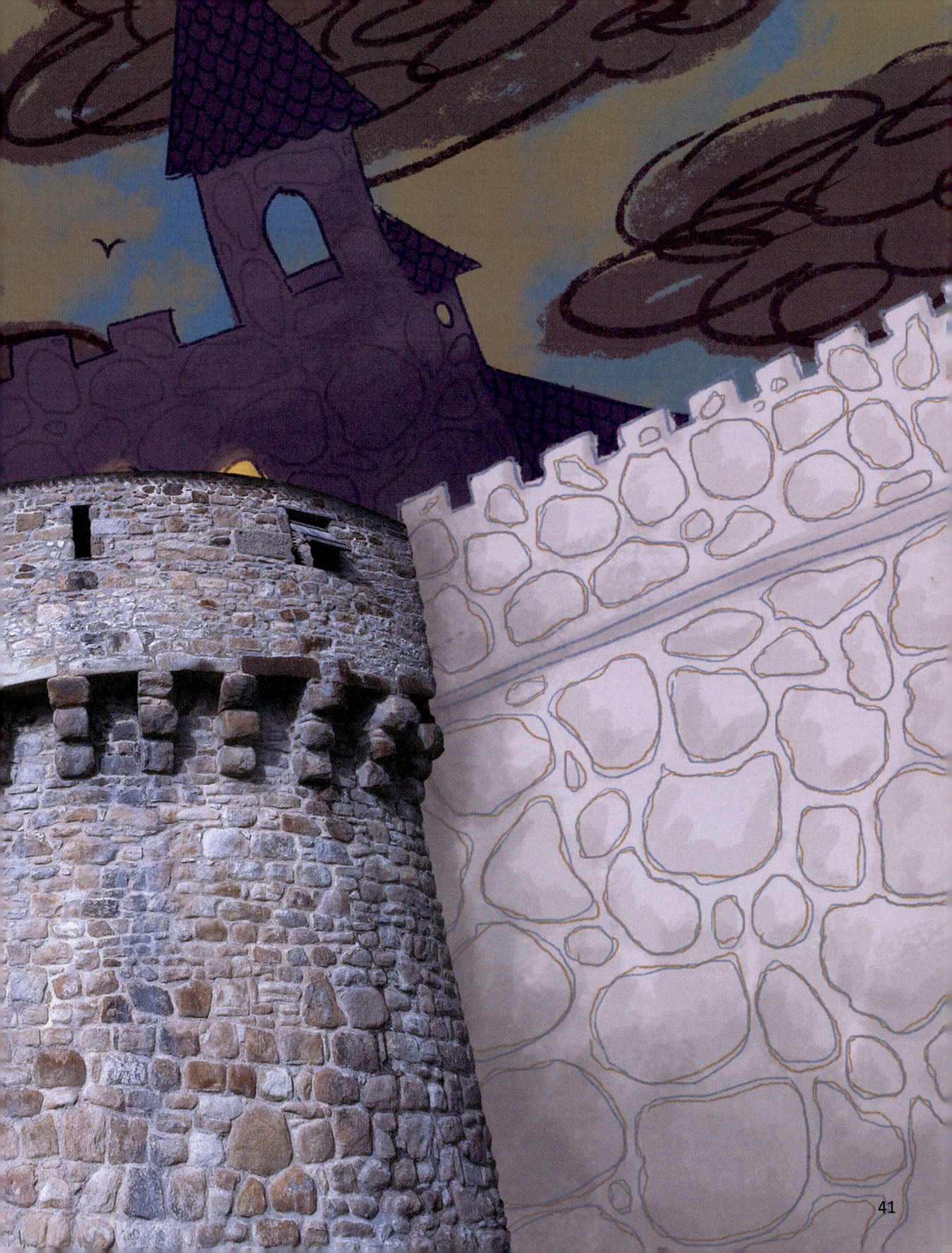

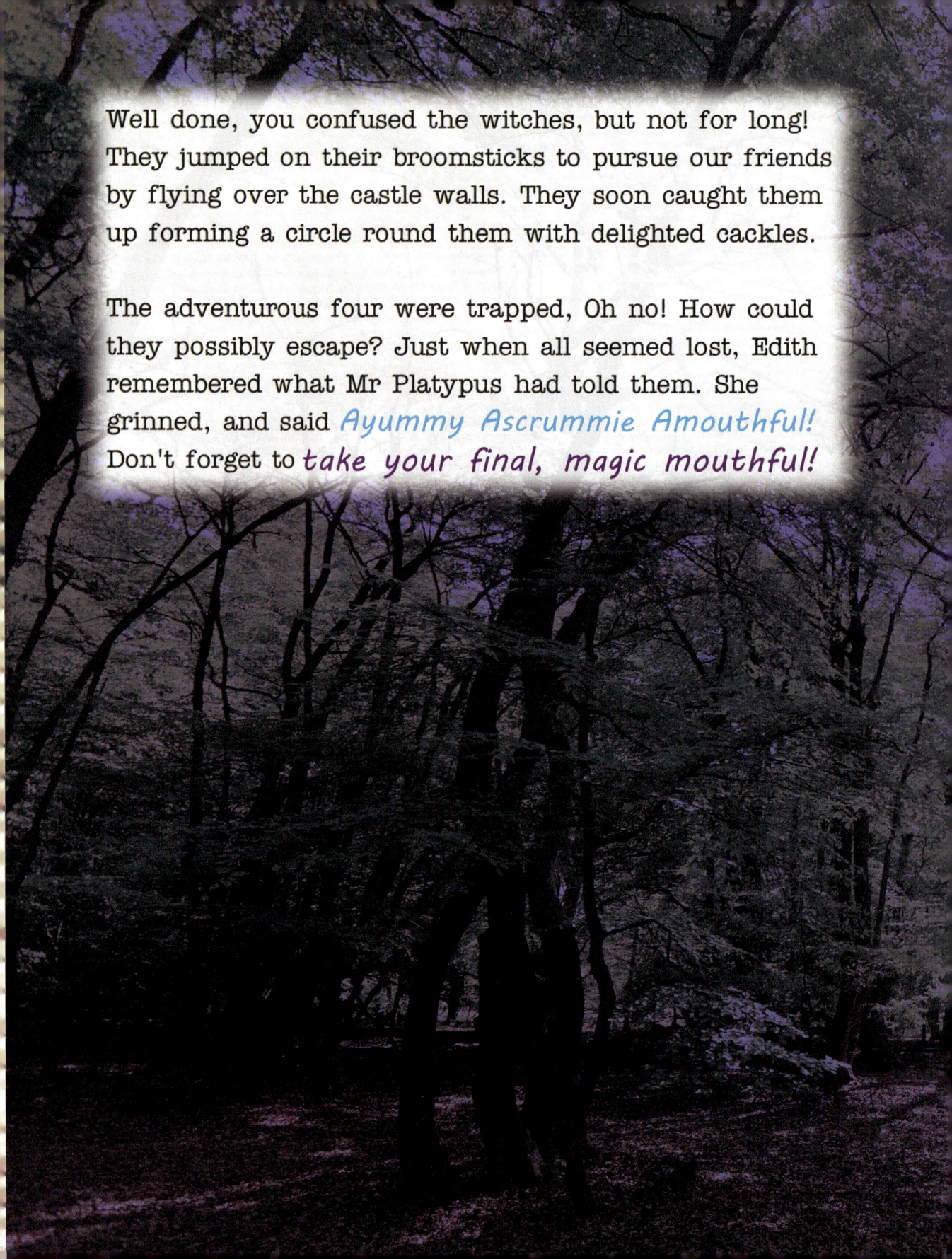

Well done, you confused the witches, but not for long! They jumped on their broomsticks to pursue our friends by flying over the castle walls. They soon caught them up forming a circle round them with delighted cackles.

The adventurous four were trapped, Oh no! How could they possibly escape? Just when all seemed lost, Edith remembered what Mr Platypus had told them. She grinned, and said *Ayummy Ascrummie Amouthful!* Don't forget to *take your final, magic mouthful!*

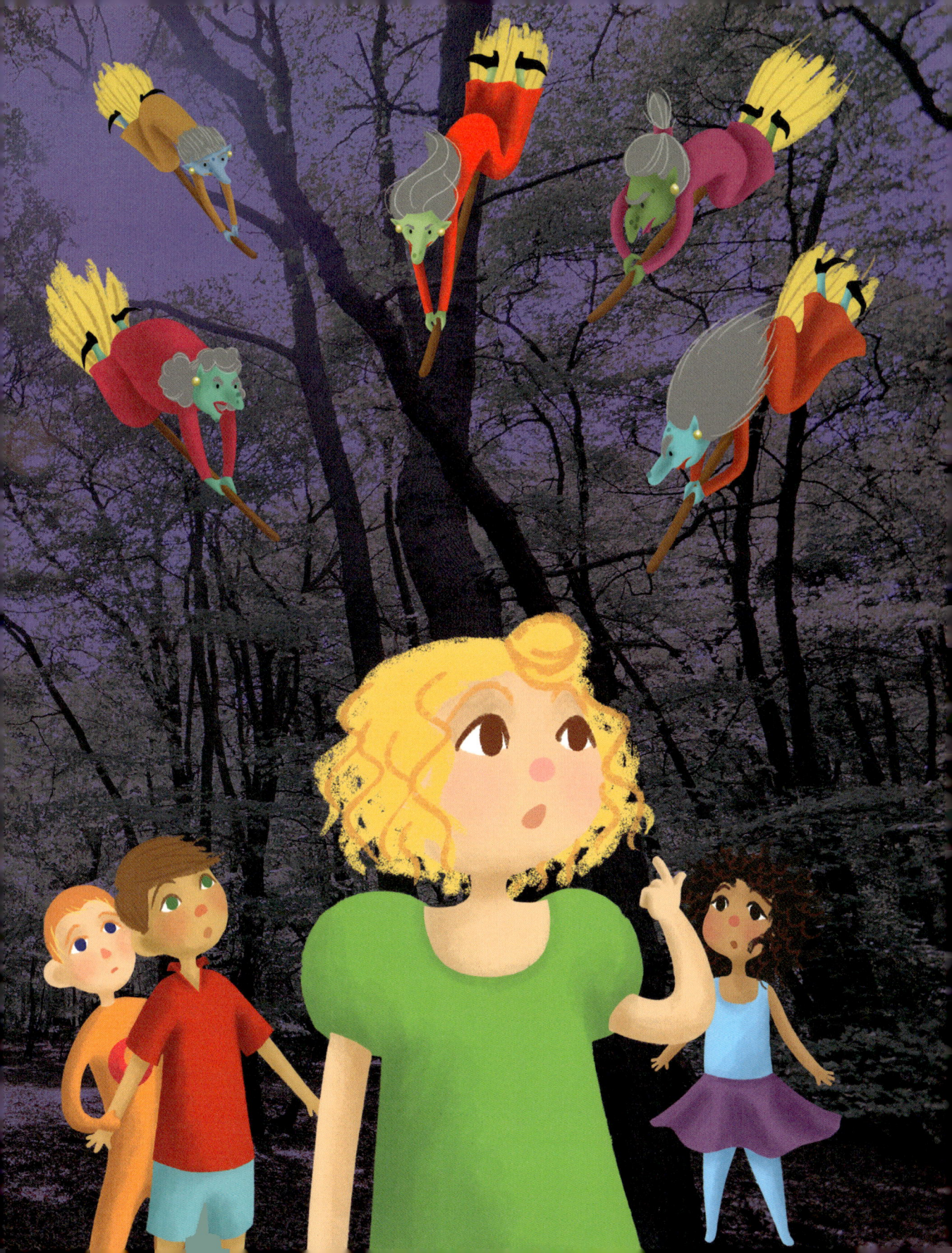

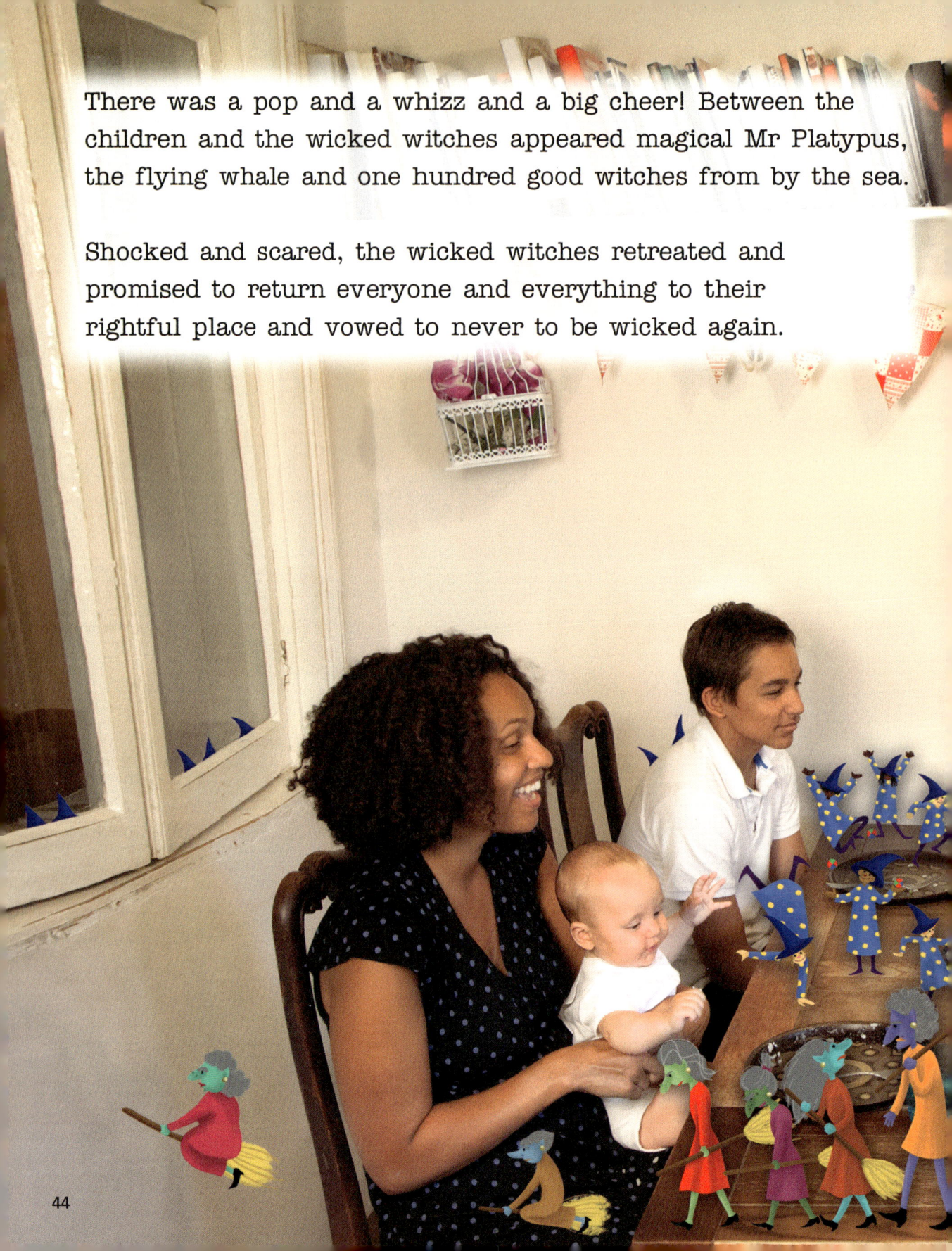

There was a pop and a whizz and a big cheer! Between the children and the wicked witches appeared magical Mr Platypus, the flying whale and one hundred good witches from by the sea.

Shocked and scared, the wicked witches retreated and promised to return everyone and everything to their rightful place and vowed to never to be wicked again.

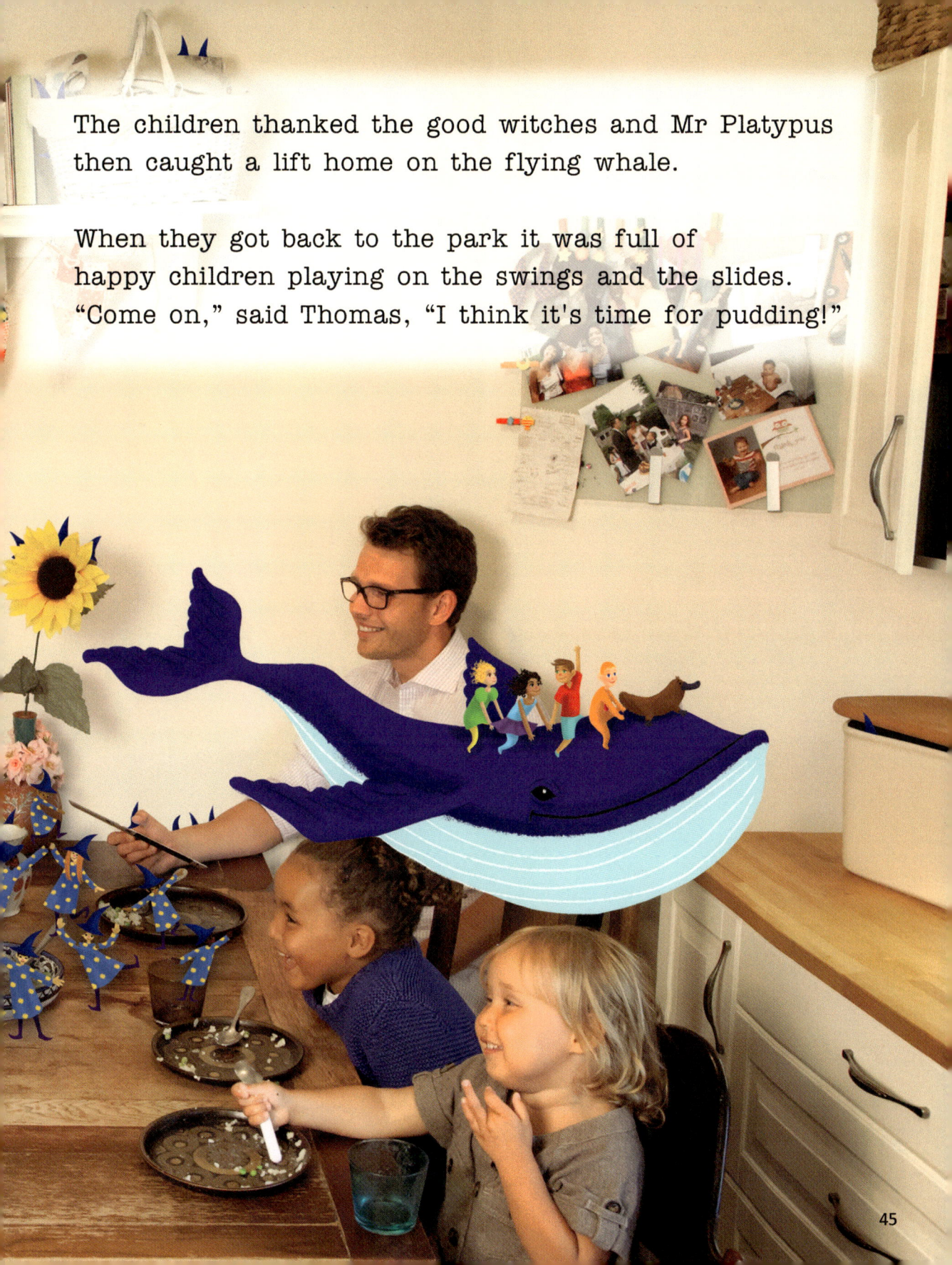

The children thanked the good witches and Mr Platypus then caught a lift home on the flying whale.

When they got back to the park it was full of happy children playing on the swings and the slides. "Come on," said Thomas, "I think it's time for pudding!"

Hints And Tips

Every child is unique and will respond to **Take Another Mouthful** stories in their own way.

Here are some *top tips* we would like to share which we hope might enhance the experience.

1. We have found the stories work best for our kids when we sit and eat with them. We think it brings us to their level and it's easier for everyone to relax and enjoy.

2. We have based our stories on teaspoon-sized mouthfuls and never endorse over-eating. We tend to focus on whether our children are full, not whether they have 'cleared their plate.'

We have posted helpful links to portion size tips at www.takeanothermouthful.com

3. The stories have been written so that we can pause at anytime, but if our children are full and still want to hear the end – we just leave out the take another mouthfuls and finish the story.

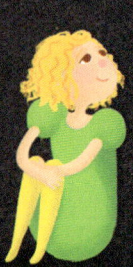

4. We try to be supportive and use positive affirmations if our children won't eat at all. We tell them that there is no pressure to eat however it is always good to try!

5. We always leave new and challenging food textures and tastes until the children are familiar and engaged with the stories. This way they are more likely to at least try!

6. These stories can be told anywhere we find they work great for us when we sit around our dinner table.

7. We try to make mealtimes special and something different. We switch the TV off and focus on our children.

8. When reading these stories to our friend's kids, we found they responded really well when we substituted the characters names for theirs. They really felt part of the story!

9. We bring out our playful side! Joining in, playing along and taking mouthfuls with the kids really helps.

About The Author

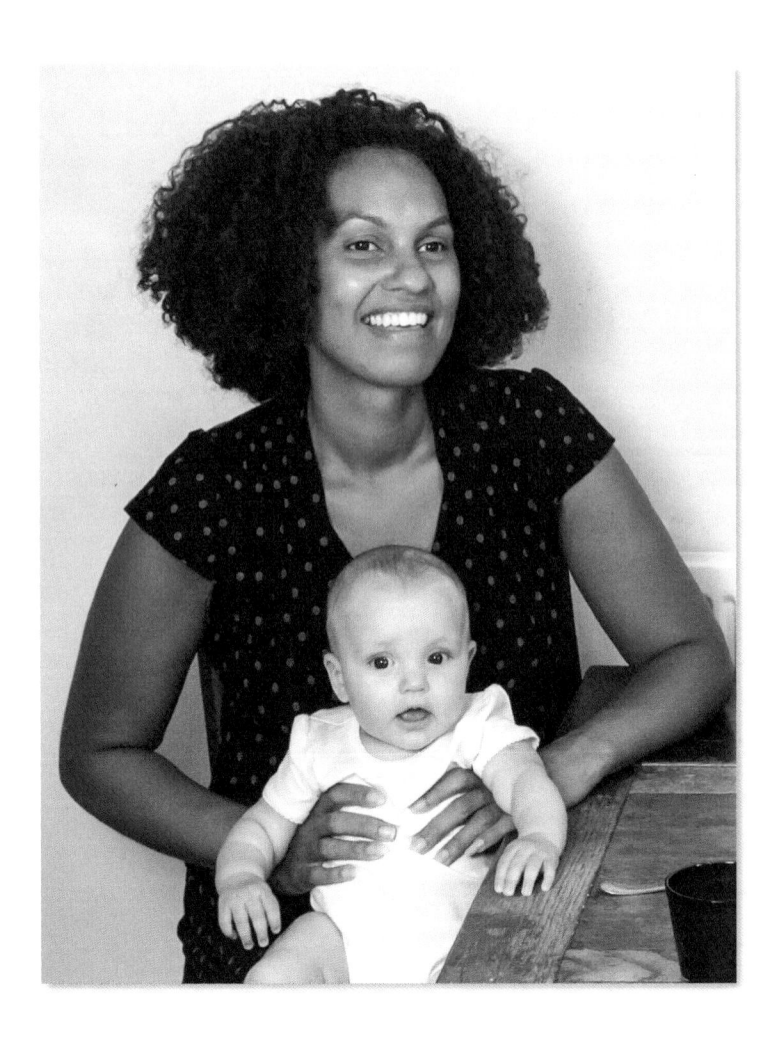

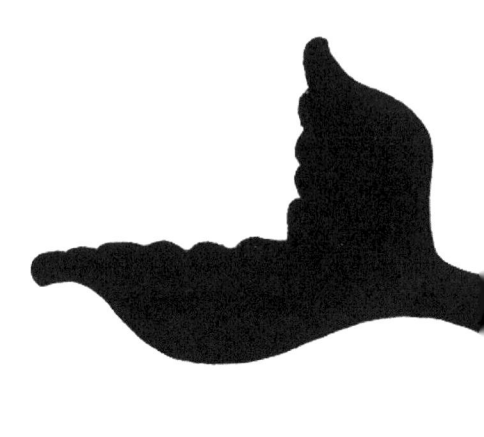

Sarah Gregory is a married full time mum with four children aged from toddler to teenager! Through her experiences she found current gaps in support for parents who were struggling with stressful mealtimes caused by fussy eating and today's busy lifestyle.

Sarah has found that many families as well as her own have faced challenges with fussy eating and finding quality time to read with their children, taking the fun out of mealtimes. Sarah married these with her husband's age-old family tradition of telling stories at mealtimes.

And so Take Another Mouthful was born! A parental tool based around a collection of adventure stories in which her children are her inspiration and a drive to make all mealtimes fun.

The Take Another Mouthful stories help her to spend quality time with her children and keep mealtimes fun and engaging. Now she wants to share the magical experience with you!

Create quality time around your dinner table and help banish the stress of fussy eating. Take Another Mouthful stories create fun family mealtimes.

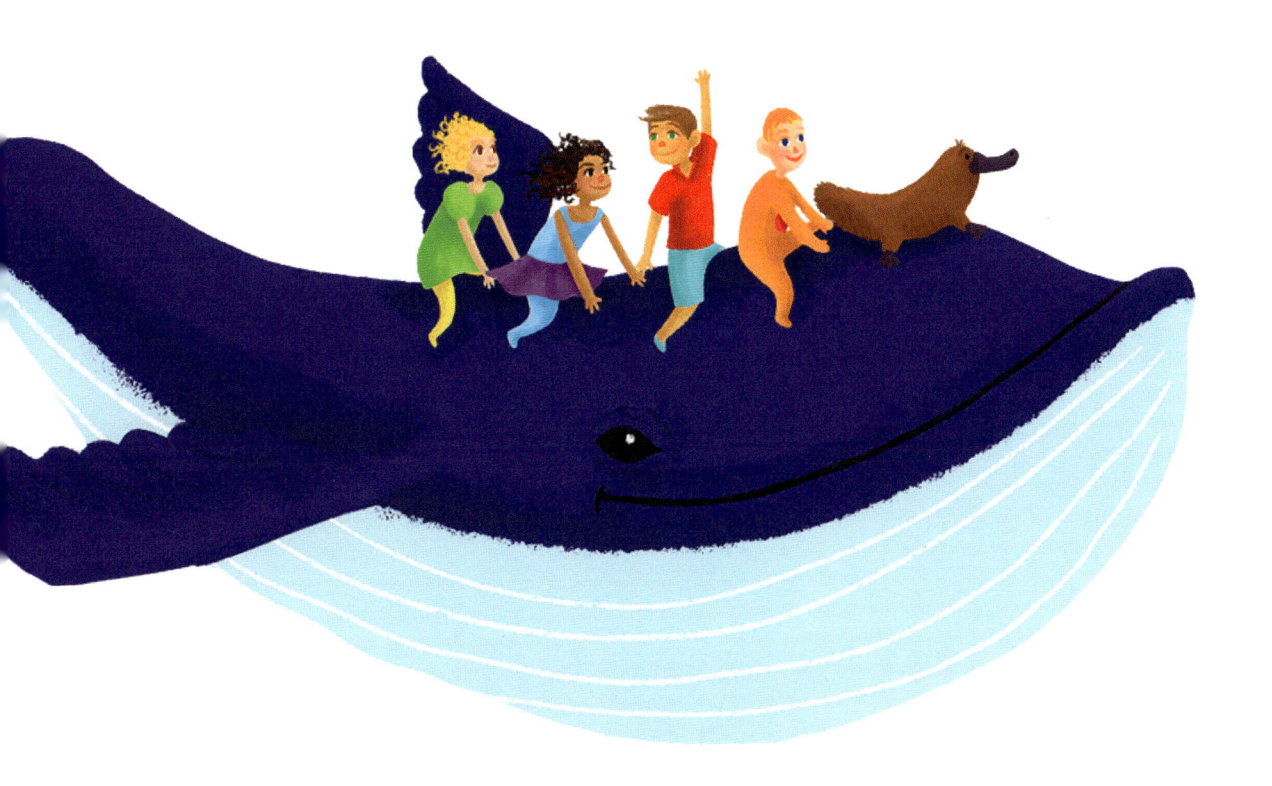

For more information about **Take Another Mouthful**
Website: **www.takeanothermouthful.com**
Facebook: **www.facebook.com/TakeAnotherMouthful**
Twitter: **@TakeAnotherM** and join our debate **#Storiesatmealtimes**

Lightning Source UK Ltd.
Milton Keynes UK
UKIC01n0757250914
239147UK00005B/19